Health Information Technology for Child and Adolescent Psychiatry

Editors

BARRY SARVET
JOHN TOROUS

CHILD AND ADOLESCENT PSYCHIATRIC CLINICS OF NORTH AMERICA

www.childpsych.theclinics.com

Consulting Editor
HARSH K. TRIVEDI

January 2017 • Volume 26 • Number 1

ELSEVIER

1600 John F. Kennedy Boulevard • Suite 1800 • Philadelphia, Pennsylvania, 19103-2899

http://www.theclinics.com

CHILD AND ADOLESCENT PSYCHIATRIC CLINICS OF NORTH AMERICA Volume 26, Number 1
January 2017 ISSN 1056–4993, ISBN-13: 978-0-323-48256-1

Editor: Lauren Boyle
Developmental Editor: Kristen Helm

Child and Adolescent Psychiatric Clinics of North America (ISSN 1056-4993) is published quarterly by Elsevier Inc., 360 Park Avenue South, New York, NY 10010-1710. Months of issue are January, April, July, and October. Business and Editorial Offices: 1600 John F. Kennedy Boulevard, Suite 1800, Philadelphia, PA 19103-2899. Periodicals postage paid at New York, NY and additional mailing offices. Subscription prices are $316.00 per year (US individuals), $566.00 per year (US institutions), $100.00 per year (US students), $367.00 per year (Canadian individuals), $688.00 per year (Canadian institutions), $200.00 per year (Canadian students), $439.00 per year (international individuals), $688.00 per year (international institutions), and $200.00 per year (international students). International air speed delivery is included in all *Clinics* subscription prices. All prices are subject to change without notice. **POSTMASTER:** Send address changes to *Child and Adolescent Psychiatric Clinics of North America*, Elsevier Health Sciences Division, Subscription Customer Service, 3251 Riverport Lane, Maryland Heights, MO 63043. **Customer Service: 1-800-654-2452 (U.S. and Canada); 314-447-8871 (outside U.S. and Canada). Fax:** 314-447-8029. **E-mail:** JournalsCustomer Service-usa@elsevier.com **(for print support) or** journalsonlinesupport-usa@elsevier.com **(for online support).**

Reprints. For copies of 100 or more of articles in this publication, please contact the Commercial Reprints Department, Elsevier Inc., 360 Park Avenue South, New York, New York 10010-1710 Tel.: 212-633-3874; Fax: 212-633-3820, E-mail: reprints@elsevier.com.

Child and Adolescent Psychiatric Clinics of North America is covered in *MEDLINE/PubMed (Index Medicus), ISI, SSCI, Research Alert, Social Search, Current Contents,* and *EMBASE/Excerpta Medica.*

Contributors

CONSULTING EDITOR

HARSH K. TRIVEDI, MD, MBA
President and Chief Executive Officer, Sheppard Pratt Health System; Clinical Professor and Vice Chair of Psychiatry, University of Maryland School of Medicine, Baltimore, Maryland

CONSULTING EDITOR EMERITUS

ANDRÉS MARTIN, MD, MPH

FOUNDING CONSULTING EDITOR

MELVIN LEWIS, MBBS, FRCPSYCH, DCH

EDITORS

BARRY SARVET, MD
Chair, Department of Psychiatry, Baystate Health; Professor and Chair of Psychiatry, The University of Massachusetts Medical School-Baystate, Springfield, Massachusetts

JOHN TOROUS, MD
Division of Clinical Informatics; Department of Psychiatry, Beth Israel Deaconess Medical Center, Harvard Medical School, Boston, Massachusetts

AUTHORS

CHRISTOPHER ARCHANGELI, MD
Child and Adolescent Psychiatry Fellow, Department of Psychiatry, University of Vermont, Burlington, Vermont

CHRISTY BENSON, BA
Senior System Analyst, Information Technology Services, University of Utah, Salt Lake City, Utah

SHARON CAIN, MD
Professor, Psychiatry & Behavioral Sciences Department, University of Kansas Medical Center, Kansas City, Kansas

MILTON CHEN, PhD
VSee, San Jose, California

SARA COFFEY, DO
Assistant Professor, Department of Psychiatry, Oklahoma State University School of Community Medicine, Tulsa, Oklahoma

ALISON M. DARCY, PhD
Instructor, Department of Psychiatry and Behavioral Sciences, Stanford School of Medicine, Stanford, California

SHIH YEE-MARIE TAN GIPSON, MD
Department of Psychiatry, Boston Children's Hospital, Harvard Medical School, Boston, Massachusetts

THOMAS GUTHEIL, MD
Department of Psychiatry, Beth Israel Deaconess Medical Center, Harvard Medical School, Boston, Massachusetts

RASHAD HARDAWAY, MD
Department of Psychiatry and Behavioral Medicine, Seattle Children's Hospital, Seattle, Washington

ERNEST JEREMY KENDRICK, MD
Assistant Professor, Department of Psychiatry, University of Utah School of Medicine, Salt Lake City, Utah

JUNG WON KIM, MD
Department of Psychiatry, Boston Children's Hospital, Harvard Medical School, Boston, Massachusetts

ROBERT KITTS, MD
Department of Psychiatry, Harvard Medical School, Boston, Massachusetts

RAJEEV KRISHNA, MD, PhD
Child Psychiatry, Nationwide Children's Hospital, The Ohio State University Wexner Medical Center, Columbus, Ohio

JAMES LOCK, MD, PhD
Professor, Department of Psychiatry and Behavioral Sciences, Stanford School of Medicine, Stanford, California

ELENI MANETA, MD
Department of Psychiatry, Boston Children's Hospital, Harvard Medical School, Boston, Massachusetts

F. ALETHEA MARTI, PhD
Post-Doctoral Researcher, UCLA Center for Health Services and Society, Los Angeles, California

EVE-LYNN NELSON, PhD
Professor, Pediatrics Department, University of Kansas Medical Center, Kansas City, Kansas; Director, KU Center for Telemedicine and Telehealth, University of Kansas Medical Center, Fairway, Kansas

TODD E. PETERS, MD
Associate Chief of Staff, Department of Psychiatry and Behavioral Sciences; Medical Director for Inpatient Services, Vanderbilt Psychiatric Hospital; Assistant Chief Medical Informatics Officer/Customer Relationship Manager, Vanderbilt University Medical Center, Nashville, Tennessee

ADAM C. POWELL, PhD
Payer+Provider Syndicate, Boston, Massachusetts

BARRY SARVET, MD
Chair, Department of Psychiatry, Baystate Health; Professor and Chair of Psychiatry, The University of Massachusetts Medical School-Baystate, Springfield, Massachusetts

STEPHEN M. SCHUELLER, PhD
Assistant Professor, Department of Preventive Medicine, Center for Behavioral Intervention Technologies (CBITs), Northwestern University, Chicago, Illinois

SUSAN SHARP, DO
Clinical Assistant Professor, Psychiatry & Behavioral Sciences Department, University of Kansas Medical Center, Kansas City, Kansas

AH LAHM SHIN, MD
Department of Anesthesia, Boston Children's Hospital, Boston, Massachusetts

COLLEEN STILES-SHIELDS, MA, MS
Clinical Psychology Doctoral Candidate, Department of Preventive Medicine, Center for Behavioral Intervention Technologies (CBITs), Northwestern University, Chicago, Illinois

CHANIDA THAMMACHART, MA
University of New England, Biddeford, Maine

JOHN TOROUS, MD
Division of Clinical Informatics; Department of Psychiatry, Beth Israel Deaconess Medical Center, Harvard Medical School, Boston, Massachusetts

ERIK VANDERLIP, MD, MPH
Assistant Professor, Department of Psychiatry, Oklahoma State University School of Community Medicine, Tulsa, Oklahoma

EMILIA ANTONIEVNA WOBGA-PASIAH, MD, MPH
Resident, Department of Family and Preventive Medicine, University of Arkansas for Medical Sciences, Fayetteville, Arkansas

EMILY WU, MD
Harvard Longwood Psychiatry Residency Training Program; Department of Psychiatry, Beth Israel Deaconess Medical Center, Harvard Medical School, Boston, Massachusetts

LANA YAROSH, PhD
Assistant Professor, Department of Computer Science and Engineering, University of Minnesota, Minneapolis, Minnesota

BONNIE ZIMA, MD, MPH
Professor-in-Residence, Department of Psychiatry and Behavioral Sciences, David Geffen School of Medicine; Associate Director, UCLA Center for Health Services and Society, Los Angeles, California

Contents

successfully across psychiatry, psychology, and developmental medicine. The authors discuss relevant issues related to delivering telemental health, including why this modality is necessary for delivery, what models and evidence for telemental health exist, when it should be considered across legal/regulatory and ethical considerations, where telemental health services are delivered, who is involved in delivery, and how best telemental health practices may be implemented with diverse youth.

Technology has become an integral part of everyday life and is starting to shape the landscape of graduate medical education. This article reviews the use of technology in teaching child and adolescent psychiatry (CAP) fellows, and 3 main aspects are considered. The first aspect is use of technology to enhance active learning. The second aspect covers technology and administrative tasks, and the third aspect is the development of a technology curriculum for CAP trainees. The article concludes with a brief review of some of the challenges and pitfalls that have to be considered and recommendations for future research.

There is a consistent need for more child and adolescent psychiatrists. Despite increased recruitment of child and adolescent psychiatry trainees, traditional models of care will likely not be able to meet the need of youth with mental illness. Integrated care models focusing on population-based, team-based, measurement-based, and evidenced-based care have been effective in addressing accessibility and quality of care. These integrated models have specific needs regarding health information technology (HIT). HIT has been used in a variety of different ways in several integrated care models. HIT can aid in implementation of these models but is not without its challenges.

This article summarizes the current literature on clinical knowledge and practical gaps regarding the confidentiality and privacy for smartphone and connected devices in child and adolescent psychiatry and offers practical solutions and consideration for the next steps for the field. Important issues to consider include disclosure of information sharing, access privilege, privacy and trust, risk and benefit analysis, and the need for standardization. Through understanding the privacy and confidentiality concerns regarding digital devices, child and adolescent psychiatrists can guide patients and parents through informed decision-making and also help shape how the field creates the next generation of these tools.

Adam C. Powell, Milton Chen, and Chanida Thammachart

This article describes the benefits resulting from the use of mobile applications for mental health and telepsychiatry. Potential direct benefits include substitution for other forms of care, prevention of higher-acuity illness, higher rate of psychiatrist use, increased competition of services driving lower treatment costs, lower operating costs for psychiatrists, fewer missed appointments, and revenue for application developers. Potential indirect benefits include improved physical health, enhanced current and future productivity, and reduced demands on caregivers. A return on investment analysis framework is then presented as a generalized means for evaluating the return on investment of specific health care interventions.

CHILD AND ADOLESCENT PSYCHIATRIC CLINICS

FORTHCOMING ISSUES

April 2017
Transitional Age Youth and Mental Illness: Influences on Young Adult Outcomes
Adele Martel and Catherine Fuchs, *Editors*

July 2017
Early Childhood Mental Health: Advancements in Assessment and Intervention, Ages 0-6
Mini Tandon, *Editor*

October 2017
Integrated Care
Gregory K. Fritz, Tami D. Benton, and Gary Maslow, *Editors*

RECENT ISSUES

October 2016
Substance Use Disorders, Part II
Ray Chih-Jui Hsiao and Paula D. Riggs, *Editors*

July 2016
Substance Use Disorders, Part I
Ray Chih-Jui Hsiao and Leslie Renee Walker, *Editors*

April 2016
Prevention of Mental Health Disorders: Principles and Implementation
Aradhana Bela Sood and Jim Hudziak, *Editors*

AACAP Members: Please go to www.jaacap.org for information on access to the Child and Adolescent Psychiatric Clinics. *Resident* Members of AACAP: Special access information is available at www.childpsych.theclinics.com.

RELATED INTEREST

Pediatric Clinics of North America, April 2016 (Vol. 63, No. 2)
Quality of Care and Information Technology
Srinivasan Suresh, *Editor*
Available at http://www.pediatric.theclinics.com/

THE CLINICS ARE AVAILABLE ONLINE!
Access your subscription at:
www.theclinics.com

CHILD AND ADOLESCENT
PSYCHIATRIC CLINICS

Preface

The Emerging Application of Health Information Technology in Child and Adolescent Psychiatry

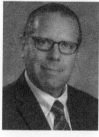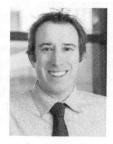

Barry Sarvet, MD   John Torous, MD
Editors

There are these two young fish swimming along and they happen to meet an older fish swimming the other way, who nods at them and says "Morning, boys. How's the water?" And the two young fish swim on for a bit, and then eventually one of them looks over at the other and goes "What the hell is water?"
—Foster Wallace, D. (2005, May). *This Is Water. Commencement speech presented at Kenyon College, Gambier, Ohio*

Like water for fish, digital technology surrounds us and has been incorporated into so many aspects of our lives that we could scarcely function without it. Until recently, child and adolescent psychiatry has operated at the margins of the health system, seemingly immune to the digital revolution occurring in other fields of medicine. With increasing recognition of the importance of mental health for overall health and well-being, child and adolescent psychiatry has "gone mainstream," and accordingly, health information technology is beginning to transform practice. Whether older or younger fish, it is important that we focus our attention on this medium that surrounds us: to reflect on the nature of the technology, to examine evidence regarding its impact upon our patients and our practice, to consider ways in which its power can be harnessed to improve the lives of our patients, and to identify and manage its attendant risks.

Several articles in this issue describe patient-facing digital technologies. For example, Schueller and his colleagues incorporate research findings regarding child-computer interaction and game theory in the consideration of online mental health treatment and virtual therapists for children and adolescents. Archangeli and

Child Adolesc Psychiatric Clin N Am 26 (2017) xiii–xv
http://dx.doi.org/10.1016/j.chc.2016.08.001
1056-4993/17/© 2016 Published by Elsevier Inc.

colleagues summarize the current state of evidence regarding the effectiveness and feasibility of smartphone apps in child and adolescent psychiatry in their systematic review. Looking at specific disorders, Darcy and Lock describe the use of technological solutions to support family-based treatment of anorexia nervosa and bulimia and summarize pilot data regarding patient experience and effectiveness. In their article regarding patient portals, Kendrick and Benson consider the opportunities and risks associated with this technology in consideration of adolescent needs for autonomy and privacy.

While patient-facing technologies offer new data and adjunctive treatments, clinician-facing technologies are equally important. Considering how clinical decision support and electronic medical records can improve care, Peters summarizes the capabilities and limitations of health information technology systems in their current iteration. Krishna summarizes evidence regarding the impact of computers in the consulting room on the patient-provider relationship and discusses potential clinical strategies for optimizing patient experience. Nelson and her colleagues review the current state of telemental health as a platform to deliver care in the context of daunting access-to-care challenges. Gipson and colleagues explore novel territory in reviewing advances in the use of technology to support education and training in child and adolescent psychiatry and in summarizing elements of a proposed technology curriculum for child psychiatry fellows.

The final three articles in the issue address overarching and systems level issues pertaining to the use of health information technology in the field of child and adolescent psychiatry. Coffey and colleagues describe the use of health information technology for the integration of child psychiatry in primary care and population health. Wu and colleagues provide a sobering warning and call to action regarding the current lack of appropriate standards for privacy and confidentiality in the context of the rapid proliferation of mobile health applications in the children's mental health field. Finally, Powell and colleagues consider the economics of health information technology for the field and consider how we can begin to measure value and sustainability.

Across the generational divide, most child and adolescent psychiatrists lag behind their patients in the comfort, facility, and trust in digital technology. Inexorable technological progress, bolstered by cultural and commercial forces, will likely continue to drive rapid advancement in the use of health information technology tools in child and adolescent psychiatry practice. It will be important to balance our exuberance regarding the promise of these tools against the need to systematically study their clinical ramifications. The articles in this issue clearly demonstrate early progress in this work: describing the use of these tools, summarizing available evidence, but most importantly, framing questions that need to be studied further.

Barry Sarvet, MD
Department of Psychiatry
Baystate Health
The University of Massachusetts Medical School-Baystate
759 Chestnut Street, WG703
Springfield, MA 01199, USA

John Torous, MD
Division of Clinical Informatics
Department of Psychiatry
Beth Israel Deaconess Medical Center
Harvard Medical School
330 Brookline Avenue
Boston, MA 02215, USA

E-mail addresses:
barry.sarvet@umassmed.edu (B. Sarvet)
jtorous@bidmc.harvard.edu (J. Torous)

Online Treatment and Virtual Therapists in Child and Adolescent Psychiatry

Stephen M. Schueller, PhD[a],*, Colleen Stiles-Shields, MA, MS[a], Lana Yarosh, PhD[b]

KEYWORDS

- Treatment • Children • eHealth/mhealth • Design

KEY POINTS

- Effective online and virtual therapies have been developed and evaluated for children and adolescents for a variety of mental and behavioral health conditions.
- Children and adolescents have unique capabilities and interests with regards to technology-based interventions that make the design of these treatments for these populations especially important.
- Future interventions should incorporate end user input early in the development process to design usable and impactful interventions for these populations.

INTRODUCTION

The need for mental health services among children and adolescents is extremely high. Estimates suggest that the 1-year prevalence of any mental disorder among those aged 13 to 17 years is 40.3%.[1] Furthermore, youth experience high rates of recurrence, suggesting that if left untreated, even symptoms that decrease over time are likely to return. Unfortunately, most youth who need services do not receive them, with only 20% of youth meeting cutoff points on mental health screening questionnaires receiving services.[2] Those who do receive services most often receive them in education settings, followed by specialty mental health services and primary care.[3] Several reasons contribute to this problem, including an insufficient workforce that is heavily concentrated in urban areas,[4] lack of knowledge and stigma toward mental

Disclosure Statement: S.M. Schueller is supported by a grant from NIMH (K08 MH102336, PI: S.M. Schueller), C. Stiles-Shields is supported by a grant from NIMH (F31 MH106321, PI: C. Stiles-Shields).
[a] Department of Preventive Medicine, Center for Behavioral Intervention Technologies (CBITs), Northwestern University, 750 North Lake Shore Drive, Chicago, IL 60611, USA; [b] Department of Computer Science and Engineering, University of Minnesota, 200 Union Street, Southeast, Minneapolis, MN 55455-0159, USA
* Corresponding author.
E-mail address: schueller@northwestern.edu

health services,[5] and the costs and resources required to regularly attend sessions that are necessary for proper care.[6] As a result, children and adolescents often receive either no or insufficient care.[7]

In light of this, several calls have been posed to transform mental health services and broaden the modes of treatment delivery.[8] One particularly promising pathway includes online and virtual therapies that could serve as alternatives and adjuncts to other services. Several instances of online and virtual therapies for children and adolescents exist,[9] with the majority focused on cognitive-behavioral principles. These tools expand access to services by creating low-cost, widely available resources and can be used in different settings by those with and without specialty mental health training.

The promise of online and virtual therapies can only be realized, however, if they are designed and implemented appropriately. Elsewhere, we have been warned of the danger of relying on "psychological skeuomorphs" while designing technologies.[10] "Psychological skeuomorphs" occur when aspects of traditional mental health services are maintained that are unnecessary and sometimes counterproductive to their delivery in digital mediums. In addition, an issue that is particularly critical for the use of these tools with children and adolescents is to ensure their appropriateness for these populations. Although most programs are tailored to be "age appropriate," this tailoring often happens at the content level. That is, the programs may tailor examples and reading levels for children and adolescents, but many of the same design principles and interaction styles present in adult programs remain.

In the current review, the state of the practice for online and virtual therapies is discussed, highlighting what has been done and what has been effective. Then, the authors draw on learning from the field of child-computer interaction to illustrate the unique considerations necessary for designing interactive technologies for children and adolescents. The article then concludes with some novel examples that are redefining the way online and virtual therapies are constructed and discusses implications for the future of providing mental health services to children and adolescents.

COMMON PRACTICES IN ONLINE AND VIRTUAL THERAPIES

Although several online therapy programs exist, they tend to share similar features. Many programs are provided along with some human contact or coaching because of the findings that supported programs tend to be more efficacious and used more than self-guided programs.[11] For youth, this could be a therapist, teacher, or one's parent. Programs also differ in terms of delivery platform and context. Many researched programs were developed to be completed on a desktop computer, through either CD-ROMs or a Web site. Last, the context of the program with regard to the provision of care is sometimes a replacement for traditional services and other times serves as an adjunct.

Human Support

Supported programs lose some of the scalability of self-guided programs; however, this tradeoff is seen as desirable because of the increases in efficacy and adherence. Completion rates in online treatments vary considerably, with a recent review finding values ranging from 12% to 100% with a median rate of 56%.[12] These rates tend to be much higher in supported programs.[13] In adult online therapies, support is most often provided by a clinician, facilitating the use of motivational tactics to increase use and ability to address technical and clinical issues that may arise. However, programs targeted at youth have the unique affordance that a parent, caregiver, or teacher could play the role of supporter. These individuals might not know as much about the clinical concepts, but have more knowledge about the child's behavior and context that might be helpful in the application of the material and supporting engagement. For example, research suggests that behavior change plans are viewed more positively when they are personalized to people's goals, patterns, and preferences, and that close others are better able to create such plans.[14] Furthermore, parents or teachers might be able to provide reinforcements that extend beyond the therapeutic relationship, thus further boosting adherence.

Delivery Platform

Most programs researched thus far have been designed for desktop computers and disseminated as either CD-ROMs or Web sites. This decision, however, impacts not only where children and adolescent access these programs but also how they interact with them. The predominant mode of interaction has been to structure programs in several sessions or modules in which users complete interactive lessons and didactic materials and then complete assignments to reinforce and practice the skills before moving on to the next lesson. For example, Camp Cope-A-Lot is a 12-session computerized adaptation of the Coping Cat program.[15,16] Each session takes approximately 35 minutes to complete. These sessions are completed with the assistance of a therapist and focus on skill building, exposure tasks, and rehearsal. Similarly, MoodGYM, an Internet-based program designed to prevent or decrease symptoms of depression and anxiety, uses a 5-module structure.[17] The modules are meant to be completed in a set order and cover topics including feelings, thoughts, unwarping, destressing, and relationships. This highly structured format is an effective way to teach material and to ensure that users receive core content related to the relevant behavior change techniques. However, this format is most likely not akin to the typical way children and adolescents are used to interacting with information in technological mediums, especially because they report being online "almost constantly" and typically on mobile devices.[18]

Context

Online and virtual therapies represent opportunities to broaden the portfolio of available mental health services. As such, it is useful to note that these resources might interact with the mental health system in different ways. In some instances, this might mean being used instead of traditional mental health services, either where no other services are available or when youth or parents prefer technological-based treatments. In other instances, these tools might augment traditional practices to enhance their efficacy through various means. As standalone treatments, it is worth noting that their ability to provide cost-effective, universal care makes them particularly appealing to provide a standard level of care as an entry into the mental health system. For example, a large-scale deployment of MoodGYM across 30 schools was able to reach nearly 1500 students across Australia.[17] This reach occurred with minimal setup, as project coordinators and teachers received a manual with instructions without other training or support. The program ultimately produced small to moderate reductions in symptoms of depression and anxiety, demonstrating the feasibility of such an approach.

Other programs might bring technology into the therapist's office, creating a novel form of interaction between child and therapist. These tools are often meant to enhance traditional psychotherapeutic activities. For example, SmartCAT is a child- and therapist-facing tool designed to facilitate use of psychotherapy skills outside of sessions and to provide therapists with information regarding skill use.[19] Children received a Smartphone app consisting of notifications and rewards. Therapists receive a Web portal to view information from the app. A small pilot trial of SmartCAT found high levels of engagement and acceptability. SmartCAT sent an average of 6.48 requests for complete entries related to skill per week, and patients completed 82.8% of them. These high rates of completion might be attributable to the ease of use of the system. These entries took less than 5 minutes on average to complete, and patients rated the app as highly usable.

Another approach, however, is to use virtual therapies to create completely new forms of therapeutic interactions. These interactions might open novel avenues to engage a patient, perhaps providing a medium that is more acceptable for children to interact with mental health information. A perfect example of this is Personal Investigator (PI),[20,21] an interactive computer game designed to be used in psychotherapy sessions. In PI, children sit alongside the therapist while playing the game, with the goal of game material helping to open up therapeutic discussion in the session. In a few small trials of PI, promising evidence has supported this notion in the form of increased therapeutic relationship, improved structure in session, and boosted child engagement.[21] PI's gamified approach might be particularly appealing to youth. As such, it is worth considering how technology can uniquely attract and engage children through creating programs and interactions.

LEARNING FROM CHILD-COMPUTER INTERACTION

As previously mentioned, an initial intuition in designing online and virtual therapies for children or adolescents may be to adopt an existing intervention by transitioning it to a digital device, for example, transitioning a paper journaling intervention to a mobile app.[22] This transition provides the immediate benefits of on-the-go access and historical data visualizations. However, this approach frequently overlooks the opportunity to design a novel intervention that leverages the unique capabilities of a particular technological system to engage and support children and adolescents. Unique technologies for these age groups have remained relatively unexplored; however, lessons can be applied from the domain of Child-Computer Interaction to provide guidance for designing such systems in the future.

Two main principles need to be considered in technology design: usability and user experience. In both of these, youth have different needs, skills, and motivations than adults, and it is not usually appropriate to deploy adult technology interventions with child or adolescent audiences.[23] In discussing each of these principles in later discussion, the authors provide general design guidelines and examples of child-centered technology that puts these guidelines into practice.

Usability

The principle of usability refers to the child's ability to effectively use the technology in question. In general, text-based input should be avoided, becuase children struggle with typing.[24] Voice[25] or handwriting recognition[26] may be able to solve this in the future, but current systems still struggle with interpreting children's input. Children also frequently struggle with positioning and manipulating a mouse pointer on a desired target,[27] although larger targets and other interventions may help address this challenge.[28] Touchscreen devices such as tablets or phones are better suited for children's pointing tasks, in that they allow for the direct manipulation of the digital object, and children as young as 2 have been shown to have moderate ability in this mode of interaction.[29] However, children may still struggle with unintended touch of onscreen targets and drawn gestures (eg, drag-and-drop).[30] One approach for addressing usability difficulties with digital interaction is known as embodied interaction, which focuses on supporting the child in acting on the physical world or through physical objects.[31] Technologies that integrate tangible, rather than mouse-based interactions have been shown to support both better problem-solving and collaboration in children.[32] Children can accomplish complex tasks using physical objects instrumented with digital intelligence. For example, children can write a computer program without typing by assembling a wooden track where each piece corresponds with an instruction.[33] As another example, children can learn practical skills by interacting with an augmented physical object, such as a toothbrush that monitors and guides them.[34] Producers of online and virtual therapies for children should consider how usability may be improved by allowing the child to rely on known gross motor and physical manipulation skills, rather than typing or precise pointing.

User Experience

In contrast to usability, user experience refers to the child's engagement and motivation to use the technology in question. Several strategies can increase engagement and motivation. The authors highlight 3 of these strategies in later discussion: challenge and feedback, social interaction, and storytelling and self-expression.

Challenge and feedback

"Flow" is an important state for which to design, because it is an indication of high levels of engagement with the task at hand.[35] While experiencing a flow state, people report a loss of self-awareness and a feeling of being at one with the activity. It has also been shown to increase interest and affect learning performance.[36] Enhancing flow could help promote completion of longer session tasks, and smaller "microflow" interactions can incentivize people to return to shorter tasks more regularly. Challenge and feedback are key factors to achieving the optimal experience of flow.[37] Technology is uniquely suited to creating these optimal experiences through challenge and feedback, because it can adjust to the needs of a specific user to ensure that the challenge presented is appropriate to his or her skill. Two design criteria may help a technology engender an experience of flow: (1) novelty and challenge, (2) clear goals and immediate feedback.[38] Perhaps the best example of flow interaction is video games,[39] where novelty is provided through an abundance of content created for each stage of the game or new challenges introduced through game elements. Furthermore, goals and feedback are generally immediately visible in the system. Online and virtual therapies should focus on creating evolving challenges appropriate to the child's skills and providing clear feedback appropriate to the intervention goals rather than more superficial components of gamification (eg, sprites and graphical user interface elements, fantasy worlds, rewarding practice of target skills with an opportunity to play a game). These principles can serve to ensure that such efforts enhance, rather than detract, from the underlying behavior change principles.

Social interaction

Another way to increase motivation and learning is incorporating a social element into the technological intervention. One approach is in leveraging "cultural forms" for types of action that invite certain forms of social collaboration and learning. For example, integrating digital intelligence into a paper storybook encourages engaged parental involvement, as a bedtime story is a cultural form common to many cultures.[40] When designing to incorporate social learning with a parent or teacher who might be serving as a supporter, technology provides the opportunity to train the adult as an ally in helping the activity remain engaging. For example, one system helped adults and kids read together remotely through an interactive agent, which suggested questions and activities that the adult could use to engage the child.[41] When designing technology to help multiple children collaborate or socially interact with each other, a system should encourage joint attention and perspective taking.[42] To support children of various skill levels and abilities, social systems work best when incorporating appropriate levels of scaffolding or support for each child. For example, one system allowed children of mixed abilities to compete and collaborate on a digital tabletop game by adjusting the difficulty of the physical task based on each child's ability.[43] Social interaction may also be achieved asynchronously by integrating gamification elements such as leaderboards and challenges, if the data presented are actively adopted to adjust to the current skill level of each user and are consistent with the goals of the intervention.[44]

Storytelling and self-expression

The ability to share stories and express aspects of one's identity may be particularly engaging to children and teenagers and has been successfully used to support therapy,[45] literacy,[46] social skills,[47] and learning complex skills like programming.[48] Younger children may practice narrative play socially[49] or simply as a way of engaging in fantasy.[50] Older children and teenagers may tell and share stories and opinions in a performative manner, as a way of enacting their identity online.[51] In both cases, it is important to consider scaffolding not only for the act of storytelling itself but also for engagement with the perceived and real audience for the child's creation. Telling stories is inherently compelling, but only if the child feels that there is somebody listening.[50]

To summarize, technology provides an opportunity to engage and support children and adolescents in unique and powerful ways. Although youth may experience usability challenges different from those of adults, reducing reliance on text-entry and mouse-based tasks may ameliorate these issues. Instead, research shows promise in focusing on direct manipulation (eg, simple pointing on touch screens) and interaction with the physical world (eg, augmenting physical objects and environments with digital capabilities). Perhaps more importantly, technology provides opportunities to engage and motivate a child or adolescent to interact with an intervention. Three strategies for increasing engagement and motivation have shown great promise in child-computer interaction research and practice: challenge and feedback, social interaction, and storytelling and self-expression. To the extent that technology provides opportunities to integrate each of these features, it can significantly increase engagement and uptake of future online and virtual therapies for children and adolescents.

THE FUTURE OF CHILD AND ADOLESCENT ONLINE AND VIRTUAL THERAPIES

This current review highlights what is known and effective thus far in online and virtual therapies for children and adolescents. Similar to findings in the adult literature, these resources are effective for the treatment and prevention of mental health issues. Another overlap is that despite their efficacy, completion rates tend to be low, especially in the absence of human support. Much recent work in this space appears to be expanding evidence for the variety of disorders, which can be treated with this approach, finding support for diverse conditions, including depression,[52] anxiety,[53] chronic pain,[54] encopresis,[55] and smoking cessation.[56] However, the authors argue that new interventions should not merely look to transport programs to new populations in terms of disorder or age range. Instead, innovative technological resources should be inspired by the behavior change principles underlying empirically supported treatments. The authors offer a few promising examples from varying sources as potential guideposts for the future of online and virtual therapies.

Social networking and messaging apps are increasingly growing in popularity and use, especially among children and adolescent populations. People, especially teens, report being on these platforms nearly constantly.[18] Leveraging social networks and peer interactions to create content for online and virtual therapies could open up new avenues for interventions and drive engaging platforms. Furthermore, as noted, social interaction can promote motivation and learning. One innovative example is *Panoply*, a Web-based, peer-to-peer cognitive restructuring platform designed to provide evidence-based techniques for mental health, without requiring the aid of clinical support.[57] In the *Panoply* platform, users post a negative thought, respond to others' thoughts, receive restructured responses, and get feedback on their performance. *Panoply* offers structure, training, and feedback to ensure that all interactions are aligned with the principles of cognitive restructuring. A proof-of-concept deployment of *Panoply* with adults in the general population found significant reductions in depressive symptoms and specific changes in reappraisal processes. Furthermore, *Panoply* was able to quickly and efficiently leverage the crowd to make personalized responses with an average response time of 9 minutes. Although training and supervision principles for adults might need to be altered for youth, this is a promising example of leveraging social interaction for motivational and learning purposes. Future systems that allow children and adolescents to be the drivers of new content could help create engaging, personalized, and novel interactions in online platforms.

Children and adolescents spend a significant amount of their leisure time engaged in fantasy play and other games. This tendency links with the notion of storytelling and self-expression previously discussed. As such, several attempts have been made to design games that can teach psychological skills while retaining elements that make games fun and engaging. One of the more innovative uses of game designs for mental health is that of SPARX, an interactive fantasy game based on the principles of cognitive-behavioral therapy.[58] Users navigate an avatar through a fantasy world overtaken by GNATs (Gloomy Negative Automatic Thoughts) and throughout the levels master skills such as relaxation, communication, and cognitive restructuring. A noninferiority trial of SPARX compared with treatment as usual taking place in specialty mental health practices, schools, and primary care clinics found that SPARX performed comparable to usual care and had higher rates of remission. A major challenge with games, however, is creating games that meet user expectations based on previous experience with the medium. The resources afforded to game development by traditional game studios far exceed the resources available in typical mental health intervention development. New mediums such as mobile apps might lower the bar for development of such resources but still necessitate the coordination of interdisciplinary teams with expertise in psychology, game design, and programming and development.

Concurrent advances in several technology-related areas, including virtual reality, machine learning, and natural language processing, have led to the development of "virtual humans" able to perform clinical tasks that had previously required humans. These tasks include providing health information and support, and clinical interviewing.[59] Virtual humans have an added benefit of being able to be tailored to match user characteristics. For example, children and adolescents could interact with a virtual peer who possesses a similar conversational style, but with the knowledge and skills of a seasoned clinician. These agents may be particularly useful for topic areas children are not comfortable disclosing to adults. Indeed, this method might help transition children to subsequent services when necessary. Currently, virtual humans have been most useful for highly structured tasks, such as information searches and interviewing, but advances in technology will further expand the capacities of such resources. Users with more experience and comfort with such technologies might be more likely to be comfortable with using such resources for health purposes, and virtual humans are a promising avenue for integration into future online and virtual therapies for children and adolescents.

SUMMARY

Online and virtual therapies are effective resources for addressing the mental health needs of youth. Although most empirical research addresses cognitive-behavioral–based programs delivered through CD-ROMs or Internet Web sites, new approaches continue to be developed and trialed. Indeed, the future of such techniques is limited only by the imagination and drive of those working in this space. Clinical practitioners could benefit from learning more about these resources that complement or extend their efforts. The authors have outlined several considerations that are relevant to the design of future resources aimed toward youth and highlight that usability and user engagement concerns for these populations differ significantly from those raised when designing for adult populations. Innovative therapies incorporating social networking, games, and virtual humans appear to be poised to make a major contribution to this area in the near future. Although these treatments may be familiar to mental health experts in terms of the core clinical skills they promote, it is hoped that the nature and style of interactions will leverage the unique affordances of the technological mediums they use. Engagement with online treatments and virtual therapists has the potential to successfully expand the mental health options available to curb the burden of mental health needs in children and adolescents.

REFERENCES

1. Kessler RC, Avenevoli S, Costello EJ, et al. Prevalence, persistence, and sociodemographic correlates of DSM-IV disorders in the National Comorbidity Survey replication adolescent supplement. Arch Gen Psychiatry 2012;69(4): 372–80.
2. Kataoka SH, Zhang L, Wells KB. Unmet need for mental health care among US children: variation by ethnicity and insurance status. Am J Psychiatry 2002; 159(9):1548–55.
3. Farmer EM, Burns BJ, Phillips SD, et al. Pathways into and through mental health services for children and adolescents. Psychiatr Serv 2003;54(1):60–6.
4. Cummings JR, Wen H, Druss BG. Improving access to mental health services for youth in the United States. JAMA 2013;309(6):553–4.
5. Clement S, Schauman O, Graham T, et al. What is the impact of mental health-related stigma on help-seeking? A systematic review of quantitative and qualitative studies. Psychol Med 2015;45(1):11–27.
6. Salloum A, Johnco C, Lewin AB, et al. Barriers to access and participation in community mental health treatment for anxious children. J Affect Disord 2016; 196:54–61.
7. Merikangas KR, He JP, Burstein M, et al. Service utilization for lifetime mental disorders in U.S. adolescents: results of the National Comorbidity Survey-adolescent supplement (NCS-A). J Am Acad Child Adolesc Psychiatry 2011; 50:32–45.
8. Kazdin AE, Blase S. Rebooting psychotherapy research and practice to reduce the burden of mental illness. Perspect Psychol Sci 2011;6(1):21–37.

9. Rooksby M, Elouafkaoui P, Humphris G, et al. Internet-assisted delivery of cognitive behavioural therapy (CBT) for childhood anxiety: systematic review and meta-analysis. J Anxiety Disord 2015;29:83–92.

10. Schueller SM, Muñoz RF, Mohr DC. Realizing the potential of behavioral intervention technologies. Curr Dir Psychol Sci 2013;22(6):478–83.

11. Spek V, Cuijpers P, Nyklicek I, et al. Internet-based cognitive behaviour therapy for symptoms of depression and anxiety: a meta-analysis. Psychol Med 2007; 37(3):319–28.

12. Waller R, Gilbody S. Barriers to the uptake of computerized cognitive behavioural therapy: a systematic review of the quantitative and qualitative evidence. Psychol Med 2009;39(5):705–12.

13. van Ballegooijen W, Cuijpers P, van Straten A, et al. Adherence to Internet-based and face-to-face cognitive behavioural therapy for depression: a meta-analysis. PLoS One 2014;9(7):e100674.

14. Agapie E, Colusso L, Munson SA, et al. PlanSourcing: generating behavior change plans with friends and crowds. In: Proceedings of the 19th ACM Conference on Computer-Supported Cooperative Work & Social Computing. New York: ACM; 2016. p. 119–33. Available at: http://dl.acm.org/citation.cfm?id=2819943. Accessed June 3, 2016.

15. Khanna MS, Kendall PC. Computer-assisted CBT for child anxiety: the coping cat CD-ROM. Cogn Behav Pract 2008;15(2):159–65.

16. Kendall PC, Hedtke KA. Cognitive-behavioral therapy for anxious children: therapist manual. Philadelphia: Workbook Pub; 2006.

17. Calear AL, Christensen H, Mackinnon A, et al. The YouthMood project: a cluster randomized controlled trial of an online cognitive behavioral program with adolescents. J Consult Clin Psychol 2009;77(6):1021–32.

18. Lenhart A. Teen, social media and technology overview. Pew Res Cent. Available at: http://www.pewinternet.org/files/2015/04/PI_TeensandTech_Update2015_0409151.pdf. Accessed June 3, 2016.

19. Pramana G, Parmanto B, Kendall PC, et al. The SmartCAT: an m-health platform for ecological momentary intervention in child anxiety treatment. Telemed J E Health 2014;20(5):419–27.

20. Coyle D, Matthews M, Sharry J, et al. Personal Investigator: a therapeutic 3D game for adolescent psychotherapy. J Interact Technol Smart Educ 2005;2(2):73–88.

21. Coyle D, Doherty G, Sharry J. An evaluation of a solution focused computer game in adolescent interventions. Clin Child Psychol Psychiatry 2009;14(3):345–60.

22. Matthews M, Doherty G. In the mood: engaging teenagers in psychotherapy using mobile phones. In: Proceedings of the SIGCHI Conference on Human Factors in Computing Systems. New York: ACM; 2011. p. 2947–56. Available at: http://doi.org/10.1145/1978942.1979379. Accessed June 3, 2016.

23. Hourcade JP. Child-computer interaction. 1st edition. Iowa City (IA): CreateSpace; 2015.

24. Druin A, Foss E, Hatley L, et al. How children search the Internet with keyword interfaces. In: Proceedings of the 8th International Conference on Interaction Design and Children. New York: ACM; 2009. p. 89–96. Available at: http://doi.org/10.1145/1551788.1551804. Accessed June 3, 2016.

25. Lovato S, Piper AM. "Siri, is this you?": understanding young children's interactions with voice input systems. In: Proceedings of the 14th International Conference on Interaction Design and Children. New York: ACM; 2015. p. 335–8. Available at: http://doi.org/10.1145/2771839.2771910. Accessed June 3, 2016.

26. Read JC, MacFarlane S, Gregory P. Requirements for the design of a handwriting recognition based writing interface for children. In: Proceedings of the 2004 Conference on Interaction Design and Children: Building a Community. New York: ACM; 2004. p. 81–7. Available at: http://doi.org/10.1145/1017833.1017844. Accessed June 3, 2016.

27. Crook C. Young children's skill in using a mouse to control a graphical computer interface. Comput Educ 1992;19(3):199–207.

28. Hourcade JP, Perry KB, Sharma A. PointAssist: helping four year olds point with ease. In: Proceedings of the 7th International Conference on Interaction Design and Children. New York: ACM; 2008. p. 202–9. Available at: http://doi.org/10.1145/1463689.1463757. Accessed June 3, 2016.

29. Hourcade JP, Mascher SL, Wu D, et al. Look, my baby is using an iPad! An analysis of YouTube videos of infants and toddlers using tablets. In: Proceedings of the 33rd Annual Conference on Human Factors in Computing Systems. New York: ACM; 2015. p. 1915–24. Available at: http://dl.acm.org/citation.cfm?id=2702266. Accessed June 3, 2016.

30. Anthony L, Brown Q, Nias J, et al. Interaction and recognition challenges in interpreting children's touch and gesture input on mobile devices. In: Proceedings of the 2012 ACM International Conference on Interactive Tabletops and Surfaces. New York: ACM; 2012. p. 225–34. Available at: http://doi.org/10.1145/2396636.2396671. Accessed June 3, 2016.

31. Antle AN. Research opportunities: embodied child–computer interaction. Int J Child Comput Interact 2013;1(1):30–6.

32. Antle AN, Droumeva M, Ha D. Hands on what?: comparing children's mouse-based and tangible-based interaction. In: Proceedings of the 8th International Conference on Interaction Design and Children. New York: ACM; 2009. p. 80–8. Available at: http://doi.org/10.1145/1551788.1551803. Accessed June 3, 2016.

33. Horn MS, Crouser RJ, Bers MU. Tangible interaction and learning: the case for a hybrid approach. Pers Ubiquitous Comput 2012;16(4):379–89.

34. Chang Y-C, Lo J-L, Huang C-J, et al. Playful toothbrush: ubicomp technology for teaching tooth brushing to kindergarten children. In: Proceedings of the SIGCHI Conference on Human Factors in Computing Systems. New York: ACM; 2008. p. 363–72. Available at: http://doi.org/10.1145/1357054.1357115. Accessed June 3, 2016.

35. Csikszentmihalyi M. Finding flow: the psychology of engagement with everyday life. New York: Basic Books; 1997.

36. O'Keefe P, Linnenbrink-Garcia L. The role of interest in optimizing performance and self-regulation. J Exp Soc Psychol 2014;53:70–8.

37. Csikszentmihalyi M. Flow: the psychology of optimal experience. New York: Harper Perennial Modern Classics; 2008.

38. Chen J. Flow in games (and everything else). Commun ACM 2007;50(4):31–4.

39. Cowley B, Charles D, Black M, et al. Toward an understanding of flow in video games. Computer in Entertainment 2008;6(2):1–27.

40. Horn MS, AlSulaiman S, Koh J. Translating Roberto to Omar: computational literacy, stickerbooks, and cultural forms. In: Proceedings of the 12th International Conference on Interaction Design and Children. New York: ACM; 2013. p. 120–7. Available at: http://doi.org/10.1145/2485760.2485773. Accessed June 3, 2016.

41. Raffle H, Ballagas R, Revelle G, et al. Family story play: reading with young children (and Elmo) over a distance. In: Proceedings of the SIGCHI Conference on

Human Factors in Computing Systems. New York: ACM; 2010. p. 1583–92. Available at: http://dl.acm.org/citation.cfm?id=1753563. Accessed June 3, 2016.

42. Yarosh S, Inkpen KM, Brush AJ. Video playdate: toward free play across distance. In: Proceedings of the SIGCHI Conference on Human Factors in Computing Systems. New York: ACM; 2010. p. 1251–60. Available at: http://dl.acm.org/authorize?N91110. Accessed June 3, 2016.

43. Brederode B, Markopoulos P, Gielen M, et al. Powerball: the design of a novel mixed-reality game for children with mixed abilities. In: Proceedings of the 2005 Conference on Interaction Design and Children. New York: ACM; 2005. p. 32–9. Available at: http://doi.org/10.1145/1109540.1109545. Accessed June 3, 2016.

44. Saksono H, Ranade A, Kamarthi G, et al. Spaceship launch: designing a collaborative exergame for families. In: Proceedings of the 18th ACM Conference on Computer Supported Cooperative Work & Social Computing. New York: ACM; 2015. p. 1776–87. Available at: http://doi.org/10.1145/2675133.2675159. Accessed June 3, 2016.

45. Matthews M, Doherty G. My mobile story: therapeutic storytelling for children. In: CHI '11 Extended Abstracts on Human Factors in Computing Systems. New York: ACM; 2011. p. 2059–64. Available at: http://doi.org/10.1145/1979742.1979860. Accessed June 3, 2016.

46. Raffle H, Vaucelle C, Wang R, et al. Jabberstamp: embedding sound and voice in traditional drawings. In: Proceedings of the 6th International Conference on Interaction Design and Children. New York: ACM; 2007. p. 137–44. Available at: http://doi.org/10.1145/1297277.1297306. Accessed June 3, 2016.

47. Tartaro A. Storytelling with a virtual peer as an intervention for children with autism. SIGACCESS Access Comput 2006;84:42–4.

48. Kelleher C, Pausch R, Kiesler S. Storytelling Alice motivates middle school girls to learn computer programming. In: Proceedings of the SIGCHI Conference on Human Factors in Computing Systems. New York: ACM; 2007. p. 1455–64. Available at: http://doi.org/10.1145/1240624.1240844. Accessed June 3, 2016.

49. Yarosh S, Kwikkers MR. Supporting pretend and narrative play over videochat. In: Proceedings of the 10th International Conference on Interaction Design and Children. New York: ACM; 2011. p. 217–20. Available at: http://dl.acm.org/authorize?N91104. Accessed June 3, 2016.

50. Cassell J, Ryokai K. Making space for voice: technologies to support children's fantasy and storytelling. Pers Ubiquitous Comput 2001;5(3):169–90.

51. Yarosh S, Bonsignore E, McRoberts S, et al. YouthTube: youth video authorship on YouTube and Vine. In: Proceedings of the 19th ACM Conference on Computer-Supported Cooperative Work & Social Computing. New York: ACM; 2016. p. 1423–37. Available at: http://doi.org/10.1145/2818048.2819961. Accessed June 3, 2016.

52. Richardson T, Stallard P, Velleman S. Computerised cognitive behavioural therapy for the prevention and treatment of depression and anxiety in children and adolescents: a systematic review. Clin Child Fam Psychol Rev 2010;13(3):275–90.

53. Spence SH, Donovan CL, March S, et al. A randomized controlled trial of online versus clinic-based CBT for adolescent anxiety. J Consult Clin Psychol 2011;79(5):629–42.

54. Palermo TM, Wilson AC, Peters M, et al. Randomized controlled trial of an Internet-delivered family cognitive-behavioral therapy intervention for children and adolescents with chronic pain. Pain 2009;146(1–2):205–13.

55. Ritterband LM, Thorndike FP, Lord HR, et al. An RCT of an Internet Intervention for pediatric encopresis with one year follow-up. Clin Pract Pediatr Psychol 2013; 1(1):68–80.
56. Patten CA, Croghan IT, Meis TM, et al. Randomized clinical trial of an Internet-based versus brief office intervention for adolescent smoking cessation. Patient Educ Couns 2006;64(1–3):249–58.
57. Morris RR, Schueller SM, Picard RW. Efficacy of a web-based, crowdsourced peer-to-peer cognitive reappraisal platform for depression: randomized controlled trial. J Med Internet Res 2015;17(3):e72.
58. Merry SN, Stasiak K, Shepherd M, et al. The effectiveness of SPARX, a computerised self help intervention for adolescents seeking help for depression: randomised controlled non-inferiority trial. BMJ 2012;344:e2598.
59. Rizzo A, Shilling R, Forbell E, et al. Autonomous virtual human agents for healthcare information support and clinical interviewing. In: Luxton DD, editor. Artificial intelligence in behavioral and mental health care. San Diego (CA): Elsevier Inc; 2015. p. 53–79.

Mobile Health Interventions for Psychiatric Conditions in Children: A Scoping Review

Christopher Archangeli, MD[a],*, F. Alethea Marti, PhD[b],
Emilia Antonievna Wobga-Pasiah, MD, MPH[c],
Bonnie Zima, MD, MPH[d]

KEYWORDS

- Mobile health • mHealth • Child • Adolescent • Pediatric • Mental health

KEY POINTS

- Clinicians, entrepreneurs, and patients are considering mobile technology as a novel way to improve mental health care delivery, especially in children and adolescents who are using mobile phones at an increasingly young age.
- Commercial development of the technology seems to be outpacing the clinical research, leaving clinicians with the difficult task of understanding how to incorporate this technology into practice.
- This review of the literature identified 8 studies of mobile health (mHealth) interventions for children with mental disorders, all of which used technology designed to enhance or augment psychotherapy.
- Most studies assessed only for feasibility. Of the 2 studies that examined effectiveness using a randomized controlled trial design, there were no statistically significant differences in clinical outcomes, but sample sizes were small.
- Despite great enthusiasm and the availability of a multitude of mental health apps, few have been rigorously studied in a clinical pediatric population and none have shown reliable evidence for improved mental health outcomes.

Disclosure: The authors have no direct conflicting interest to disclose. All authors are presently engaged in the development and study of a product related to the matter presented. Any future royalties from this product will go to the University of California, not to the authors.
[a] Department of Psychiatry, University of Vermont, 1 South Prospect Street, Burlington, VT 05401, USA; [b] UCLA Center for Health Services and Society, 10920 Wilshire Boulevard, Suite 300, Los Angeles, CA 90024, USA; [c] University of Arkansas for Medical Sciences, Northwest Family Medicine Residency, 1125 North College Avenue, Fayetteville, AR 72701, USA; [d] Department of Psychiatry and Behavioral Sciences, David Geffen School of Medicine, UCLA Center for Health Services and Society, 10920 Wilshire Boulevard, Suite 300, Los Angeles, CA 90024, USA
* Corresponding author.
E-mail address: Christopher.Archangeli@uvmhealth.org

Child Adolesc Psychiatric Clin N Am 26 (2017) 13–31
http://dx.doi.org/10.1016/j.chc.2016.07.009
1056-4993/17/© 2016 Elsevier Inc. All rights reserved.

INTRODUCTION

The development and increasing affordability of smartphones have created new possibilities in integrating mental health interventions into users' everyday lives. As increasing numbers of adolescents[1] and even young children[2] start to have their own mobile devices, both application (app) developers and clinicians are realizing the potential of mobile technology to deliver care in a novel way for this younger population.

Over the past decade, mobile technology and its adaptation have progressed rapidly. Text messaging overtook phone calls as the most frequent form of communication in 2007,[3] and that same year Apple released the first iPhone. A 2015 Pew research report shows that 64% of American adults own smartphones, up from 35% in 2011, and that 62% of smartphone owners have used them to look up information about a health condition in the last year.[4] A 2015 Gallup poll reports that 81% of smartphone owners keep their phones near them almost all the time and 72% check them at least hourly.[5]

In addition, children and adolescents comprise a large proportion of frequent mobile phone users. According to recent Pew reports, the percentage of American teenagers who use smartphones has ranged between 73% and 77% since 2009.[1,6] This technology also crosses socioeconomic lines: in 2014, 61% of adolescents from low-income (<$30,000) families owned or used a smartphone, whereas 48% owned or used a tablet.[1] According to a national survey by Common Sense Media, the percentage of children 8 years old and younger who have ever used a smartphone or tablet increased from 38% in 2011 to 72% in 2013, with 17% of children using such a device daily and 28% using it weekly.[7] Children are also starting to use mobile technology at a much younger age: in 2011, 10% of children less than 2 years old had at some point in their lives used a smartphone or tablet.[7] By 2013, this number had increased to 38%, most of whom (22%) had used the device for educational games.[7]

The progression of mobile technology has spawned a novel domain of health care: mobile health (mHealth). Evidence supporting the effectiveness of mHealth interventions to change health-related behaviors among persons with chronic conditions is mixed. Positive results have been found for the use of mHealth technologies to improve smoking cessation,[8] diabetes,[9] and weight-loss.[10] However, a Cochrane Review of mHealth interventions for asthma, one of the most studied conditions in mHealth, revealed mixed, inconclusive results.[11]

Although there is some evidence for mHealth interventions for mental health conditions, such as depression[12] and bulimia,[13] there seems to be an especially pronounced disconnect between the commercial development of mobile apps for mental health and the completion of research to validate their use. A 2013 review found more than 1500 apps for depression, but only 32 published research studies on those apps.[14] In another review focused on depression apps, only 10% of the apps on the market incorporated evidence-based principles of cognitive behavior therapy (CBT) or behavioral activation.[15] Researchers even found that only 4 of the 27 mental health apps endorsed by the UK National Health Service incorporated evidence-based interventions.[16] In addition, most of the mobile apps for mental health care have been developed for and studied in adult populations.

Nevertheless, mobile technology and its adaptation to improve the care of child mental health conditions remains promising. This article thus reviews the evidence in support of mHealth interventions for use in childhood psychiatric disorders with the goal of informing clinicians regarding their potential application in practice.

METHODS
Literature Search

A scoping review was conducted of the published academic literature, modeled on the methodology developed by Arksey and O'Malley.[17] The research question guiding this review is:

What evidence exists supporting the clinical use of mHealth interventions in addressing pediatric psychiatric disorders?

The authors conducted a structured literature search of the PubMed, PsycINFO, and Scopus databases from 1/1/2005 to 3/31/2016, using keywords designed to elicit articles meeting 3 criteria:

1. Children less than 18 years old,
2. Who were diagnosed with a Diagnostic and Statistical Manual of Mental Disorders (DSM)–IV or DSM-V classified mental health disorder, and
3. Were using some sort of mHealth intervention.

Chronologic scope

A start date of 2005 was chosen in order to focus on studies that best represent present-day mobile communication technology and avoid inclusion of outdated technology that no longer exists in production. This starting date encompasses the introduction of iPhone, Android, and Windows smartphones, as well as the shift from using mobile phones predominately for voice communication to text messaging as the most ubiquitous method of mobile communication.[3] Within this fluid technological environment, it would not be helpful to present-day clinicians to examine studies about text-messaging interventions from the year 2000, when text messaging was not commonplace and not included in typical mobile phone plans.

Search terms

With the assistance of a biomedical science librarian, the authors defined the search terms to be used and identified 3 target electronic research databases (PubMed, PsycINFO, and SCOPUS) as being the most relevant for our search. Queries were crafted for each of our 3 criteria (children, mental health diagnosis, and mHealth intervention) using medical subject heading (MeSH) terms and keywords were grouped using Boolean "OR" operators. The 3 queries were combined using "AND" operators. The search excluded studies that were not written in English. The complete search algorithms are included in **Box 1**.

Manual search

In addition to the electronic database search, included studies, as well as review articles that met the criteria listed earlier, were manually searched for additional relevant studies. Using Google Scholar and/or PubMed tools, the authors looked to find whether any studies that cited included studies also met inclusion criteria. In addition, high-yield journals were searched from 2005 (or inception) to March 2016 including the *Journal of Medical Internet Research*, *JMIR Mental Health*, *JMIR Human Factors*, and *JMIR mHealth and uHealth*.

Inclusion Criteria

Age

The literature scan searched for studies with research participants aged 18 years or younger; however, studies that contained both child and adult participants were eligible for inclusion if they provided separate outcome data for all subjects less than 18 years of age. Despite this more inclusive age criterion, none of the studies

---

Box 1
Search terms

PubMed/MEDLINE

("child"[MeSH Terms] OR "adolescent"[All Fields] OR "adolescence"[All Fields] OR "child"[All Fields] OR "childhood"[All Fields] OR "children"[All Fields] OR "pediatric"[All Fields]) AND ("mental health"[All Fields] OR "mental disorder"[All Fields] OR "mental illness"[All Fields] OR "psychiatric"[All Fields] OR "psychiatry"[All Fields] OR "tic disorder"[All Fields] OR "eating disorder"[All Fields] OR "substance use disorder"[All Fields] OR "mood disorder"[All Fields] OR "conduct disorder"[All Fields] OR "oppositional defiant disorder"[All Fields] OR "ADHD"[All Fields] OR "depression"[All Fields] OR "anxiety"[All Fields] OR "autism"[All Fields] OR "mental disorders"[MeSH Terms]) AND ("mobile technology"[All Fields] OR "smart phone application" [All Fields] OR "mobile phone application" [All Fields] OR "smart phone applications" [All Fields] OR "mobile phone applications" [All Fields]OR "mobile application"[All Fields] OR "mobile applications"[All Fields] OR "mobile app"[All Fields] OR "mobile apps"[All Fields] OR "telemedicine"[MeSH Terms] OR "mhealth"[All Fields] OR "mobile health"[All Fields] OR "mobile applications"[MeSH Terms]) AND (("2005/01/01"[PDAT]: "3000/12/31"[PDAT]) AND "humans"[MeSH Terms] AND English[lang])

SCOPUS

TITLE-ABS-KEY (child* OR adolescen* OR pediatr*) AND TITLE-ABS-KEY ("mental health" OR "mental disorder" OR "mental illness" OR psychiatr* OR "eating disorder" OR "substance use disorder" OR "conduct disorder" OR "oppositional defiant disorder" OR "ADHD" OR "mood" OR "depression" OR "anxiety" OR "autism" OR "tic disorder") AND TITLE-ABS-KEY ("mobile tech*" OR "mobile app*" OR "mobile phone app*" OR "smart phone app*" OR "mhealth" OR "mobile health") AND PUBYEAR > 2004 AND (LIMIT-TO (LANGUAGE, "English"))

PsycINFO

(child* OR adolescen* OR pediatr*) AND ("mental health" OR "mental disorder" OR "mental illness" OR psychiatr* OR "eating disorder" OR "substance use disorder" OR "conduct disorder" OR "oppositional defiant disorder" OR "ADHD" OR "mood" OR "depression" OR "anxiety" OR "autism" OR "tic disorder") AND ("mobile tech*" OR "mobile app*" OR "mobile phone app*" OR "smart phone app*" OR "mhealth" OR "mobile health")

---

that were ultimately selected for review had mixed-age participant pools, and the only adult research participants were parents of target children.

Mental disorder

Studies were included if they evaluated subjects diagnosed with, or at risk for, a mental disorder defined in the DSM. Studies that assessed nonspecific mental health symptoms in a nonclinical population, such as mood symptoms in healthy subjects, were not included. In the final list of studies selected for this review, all but one involved children or adolescents who had been diagnosed with and were receiving care for a DSM-defined mental disorder: the one exception was a study of a mobile intervention designed to prevent adolescent depression.[18]

Mobile health

Studies were included if they used a mobile device as the primary method of delivering an intervention for the identified disorder, and the delivery was unique to mobile devices. Studies that were simply adaptations of face-to-face interventions were excluded (eg, a telepsychiatry treatment that simply used phones for verbal communication, or using a tablet as a replacement for paper forms during patient intake). Mobile devices were defined as generally as possible: including mobile phones, SMS (short message service) text messaging, tablets, and personal digital assistants (PDAs), but did not include computer and Web-based interventions unless they had a mobile component.

Study design criteria

Studies had to include outcome data regarding the mHealth intervention. Given the novelty of the field, outcomes such as usability, acceptance, or feasibility were considered acceptable in addition to clinical outcomes. Many articles were found describing the development and design process of a technology without any form of outcome data involving users with mental disorders, and these were excluded.

Publication types

All publication types were considered that presented novel data. Conference articles were included as well as journal articles, because the field is in early development and the technology is constantly evolving.

Autism studies

During early analysis of the search results many studies were discovered of mHealth interventions designed to help autistic patients learn social routines or to serve as augmentative and alternative communication devices. The authors made the decision to exclude these articles because the apps discussed were very different in design, use, and goals from those used for other child behavioral care, and therefore seemed less relevant to the typical child psychiatrist's area of practice. In addition, several review articles specific to this niche have already been published,[19-21] and manual review of these yielded more than double our original results. The number of new studies that were not picked up by our original search suggests that these types of interventions are inherently different from the more general mental health mobile apps that our search was designed to identify.

Screening of Results and Data Extraction

Search results were imported into the bibliographic management program Zotero. After removal of duplicate results, studies were screened by title for any obvious reasons why they did not meet inclusion criteria. The remaining studies were sequentially excluded based on age, mental disorder, mHealth intervention, and design criteria. If the reviewer was unable to determine criteria by abstract alone, the full study was reviewed. All studies were first coded by one reviewer (CA) and these results were reviewed for accuracy by a second reviewer (either FAM or EWP). In cases of disagreement, studies were discussed until consensus was reached. Articles that met full inclusion criteria were assessed and relevant data were extracted into a table (**Table 1**). At least two authors examined each article to ensure accuracy and decrease bias.

RESULTS
Literature Scan

The initial search yielded 541 total results with 466 unique results. Ninety-four studies were judged to be obviously irrelevant based on title alone. The remaining abstracts were screened for inclusion criteria as shown in **Fig. 1**. The initial screening process found 5 studies that met the inclusion criteria as well as 12 relevant review articles. Manual search of these studies and review articles led to the identification of 3

Table 1
Synopsis of included studies

	Intervention, Device, Details	Target Disorder; Role & Description of Intervention; Availability to Public	Study Design, Purpose and Length of Intervention[a]	Study Sample Details[b]	Results
Interventions for Anxiety Disorders					
De Sa & Carrico,[26] 2012 (conference article)	Mobile App Device: PDA Target User: Child (during therapy session)	Anxiety Disorders: Enhancement for cognitive behavioral therapy (CBT) for anxiety. Helps children better quantify fears and improve discussions with therapist. Patient was provided with a PDA to use during therapy (model not specified). Intervention is not available to public.	Description of app development and a pilot qualitative analysis of feasibility using direct observation, interviews, and questionnaires. No control group. Length of intervention: 1 session.	10 children (6–14 y) 5 therapists 4 parents Portugal	8 of the children were interviewed: 3 were very pleased with the experience, 5 found it easy to use, and 7 found it easier than the paper equivalent. Therapists and parents were reported to be enthusiastic about the app.

Pramana et al,[22] 2014 (journal article)	SmartCAT (Mobile App) Devices: Android phone, Web portal Target Users: Child & Therapist	Anxiety Disorders: Supplement for "Coping Cat" child CBT for anxiety disorders. The app has five components: (1) notification reminders, (2) skills coach where child earns points for completing various tasks, (3) reward bank to spend the points, (4) media library where therapist can store personalized education materials, and (5) secure messaging between patient and therapist. Patient was provided with a mobile phone. SmartCAT is listed on GooglePlay, but intervention is only available to study participants.	Qualitative analysis of app feasibility using app usage data, a user feedback form and standardized questionnaires. No control group. Length of intervention: 6-16 sessions.	9 children (9–14 y) USA	Patients rated the app as highly usable (mean = 1.7 on a 1–7 scale, with 1 = "easy"). Patients completed a weekly average of 5.36 skills coach entries out of 6.48 prompts (82% completion rate). Parents of patients said they would recommend the program to others.

(continued on next page)

Table 1
(continued)

Intervention, Device, Details	Target Disorder; Role & Description of Intervention; Availability to Public	Study Design, Purpose and Length of Intervention[a]	Study Sample Details[b]	Results
Whitesidet al,[23] 2014 (journal article)	**Mayo Clinic Anxiety Coach (Mobile App)** Device: iOS phone Target User: Child (*setup assisted by therapist*)	**OCD/Anxiety Disorders:** App for delivering CBT for anxiety disorders. Consists of 3 modules: (1) self-assessment to determine severity of anxiety, (2) education, and (3) treatment by creating "fear ladder" hierarchies and recording exposures to anxiety-provoking stimuli. One case study used the app as a stand-alone intervention for mild OCD symptoms; the other used it as an adjunct to treatment for severe OCD complicated by geographical distance. Study did not specify whether patients used their own smartphones or were provided with one. Intervention is available to public: $4.99 on iTunes.	Case study of two youth (one diagnosed as mild, the other severe). Includes usage data and qualitative interviews as well as pre-post assessment of clinical symptoms within subjects. Length of intervention varied.	2 child case studies (10 and 16 y) demographics (and possibly gender) have been changed to protect confidentiality USA	Both patients had improvement in their OCD symptoms across multiple clinician and self-report rating scales (CY-BOCS, CGI, ARS). Both patients and their parents provided positive feedback about the app, but parents were less comfortable than children in using it.

Interventions for Depressive Disorders

Kobak et al,[24] 2015 (journal article)	Mobile webpage + text messaging Devices: iPad, cellphone Target Users: Child & Therapist	Depressive Disorders: Technology enhanced CBT approach for treating adolescent depression. Intervention consists of (1) an online training tutorial for the clinician, (2) online educational materials and tools to demonstrate CBT concepts to the patient during clinical sessions, (3) patient receives daily interactive text messages on their phone and responds with recordings of their practice sessions. Study did not specify whether therapist used their own iPad or was provided with one. Text messages were sent to patient's own phone. Intervention is not available to public.	Controlled trial evaluating feasibility, user satisfaction, and effectiveness of the technology. Each participating clinician recruited 4 patients; clinicians were randomized to intervention (35 patients) or treatment as usual (30 patients) groups. Multiple rating scales were used to assess clinical outcomes. Length of intervention: 12 wk (some outcomes measured at 8 wk)	65 children (12–17 y) 66% female. 41% Caucasian; 36% African American (35 CBT + 30 TAU) 18 clinicians USA	User satisfaction was ranked 5.6 out of 7. 95% of patients said reviewing text messages with their therapist was helpful, and all said they would use text messaging in treatment again. A significant reduction in depression symptoms was found in each group. While all clinical ratings of improvement were greater for the intervention group, the difference did not reach statistical significance. Ratings of the therapeutic alliance were higher in the intervention group ($P = .001$).

(continued on next page)

Table 1
(*continued*)

Intervention, Device, Details	Target Disorder; Role & Description of Intervention; Availability to Public	Study Design, Purpose and Length of Intervention[a]	Study Sample Details[b]	Results
Matthews & Doherty,[27] 2011 (conference article)	Mobile Mood Diary (Mobile App) Device: Smartphone Target User: Child	Mood/Depressive Disorders: Patient enters self-reports of mood, sleep, and energy by filling out numerical scales and inputting into a free-text diary. App can be accessed via both phone and web. Self-report data can be graphed over time. Patient was provided with a smartphone if they did not already own a compatible device. Intervention is not publicly purchasable, but therapists interested in using the app for treatment can contact the first author.	Qualitative analysis of feasibility using direct observation, app usage data, and interviews. No control group. Length of intervention varied (7–362 d).	9 children (10–17 y) 30% female 1 parent 3 therapists Children receiving treatment in public mental health clinics. Ireland	One patient's parent independently inputted reports about her child. Length of time that patients used the app varied widely from 7–326 d. Excluding one child (who used a modified version of the app), and including the parent, mean adherence (days with entry/days used) was 66%. (*See our discussion section for problems interpreting these percentages.*) When recording an entry, participants completed 90% of the prompts. Therapist adoption was limited by technical confidence. Online graph was used successfully in sessions.

| Whittaker et al,[18] 2012 (journal article) | Multimedia text messaging + mobile website Device: Smartphone Target User: Adolescent | Depressive Disorders: CBT-informed depression prevention intervention delivered via mobile phone SMS messaging. Participants receive daily mobile phone messages with text, videos, and/or cartoon images. Messages were sent to patient's own phone. Intervention is not available to public. | RCT, double-blind, placebo controlled trial. Treatment group received CBT-based messages; control group received similar style messages (texts, videos and cartoons) with general advice. Study assessed feasibility and self-report of CBT skills via questionnaire. Length of intervention: 9 wk | 855 teens (13–17 y) (426 intervention + 429 control) 68% female. 58% European; 24% Asian; 10% Maori New Zealand | Over three-quarters of participants viewed at least half of the messages, and 38% chose to share a message with another person. 91% of the intervention group reported they would refer the program to a friend. Intervention group participants said the intervention helped them to be more positive (67%) and to get rid of negative thoughts (50.2%), significantly higher than proportions in the control group. |

(continued on next page)

Table 1
(continued)

Interventions for Other Mental Health Disorders

	Intervention, Device, Details	Target Disorder; Role & Description of Intervention; Availability to Public	Study Design, Purpose and Length of Intervention[a]	Study Sample Details[b]	Results
Jones et al,[25] 2014 (journal article)	Mobile daily surveys + video recording + text messaging Device: Smartphone Target User: Parent	Disruptive Behavior Disorders: Technology-enhanced (TE) version of Helping the Noncompliant Child (HNC), an evidence-based Behavioral Parent Training (BPT) program. Intervention includes: (1) Skill modeling video series, (2) brief daily surveys inputted via phone, (3) text message reminders, (4) video recording of home practices, (5) mid-week video calls with therapist. Parent was provided with a smartphone. Intervention is not available to public.	Controlled trial, describes development and initial pilot testing of intervention. Assesses engagement, skill generalization and behavior outcomes both between and within groups. Families were randomized to HNC or TE-HNC groups. Length of intervention: 8–12 sessions.	15 parents of children 3–8 y (7 HNC + 8 TE-HNC) Low income: <150% poverty 87% of parents were female USA	TE-HNC appeared to boost child behavior outcomes (measured using ECBI) and had large effect sizes for all outcomes, however none of these results had statistical significance (possibly due to the small sample size). Patients in the TE-HNC were more likely to attend weekly sessions, participate in mid-week calls, and complete their home practice than families in HNC.

| Pina et al,[28] 2014 (conference article) | ParentGuardian (Mobile App) Devices: Windows 8 smartphone, tablet, wearable sensor. Target User: Parent | ADHD: Technology enhancement of BPT for parents of children with ADHD. Can be used in three ways: (1) A wearable sensor measures for physiologic signs of patient stress and triggers phone reminders with tips for coping strategies in the "heat-of-the-moment." (2) Parents use the mobile app is used to access reflective strategies and input self-reports of moods. (3) A hands-free peripheral display presents image prompts without text. Parent was provided with the smartphone, sensor and peripheral display. Intervention is not available to public. | Qualitative analysis of feasibility using direct observation, app usage data, interviews, and questionnaires. No control group. Study consists of 2 phases: Week 1: parents use only the app, and receive hourly prompts. Week 2: parents use app plus sensor and receive prompts in response to sensor. Length of intervention: 2 wk | 10 parents (8 mothers) of children in grades K-12 USA | App's usefulness for learning coping strategies was rated 5.1 out of 7. Parents averaged two coping strategy prompts per evening, some of these were "obvious" false positives that parents ignored. User ratings on some aspects of the intervention decreased in phase 2, however these data are difficult to interpret. |

Abbreviations: ADHD, attention-deficit/hyperactivity disorder; ARS, Anxiety Rating Scale; BPT, behavioral parent training; CGI, Clinical Global Improvement; CY-BOCS, Children's Tale-Brown Obsessive-Compulsive Scale; ECBI, Eyberg Child Behavior Inventory; HNC, Helping the Noncompliant Child; OCD, obsessive-compulsive disorder; RCT, randomized controlled trial; SMS, short message service; TAU, treatment as usual; TE, technology enhanced.

[a] Length of intervention is listed as number of sessions, if study did not detail the actual time interval between sessions.
[b] This column includes patient gender, ethnicity and family SES/income if information was listed in the article.

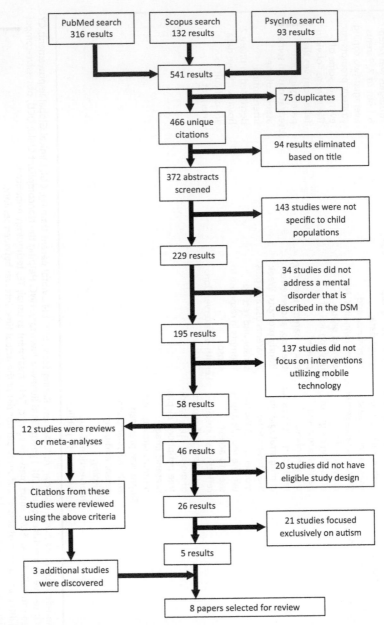

Fig. 1. The search results and screening process.

more studies that met inclusion criteria for a total of 8 included studies (see **Table 1**). The 8 studies were published between 2011 and 2015, 5 in journal articles[18,22–25] and 3 as conference articles.[26–28] Five were conducted in the United States.[22–25,28] Three articles addressed mood/depression,[22,23,26] 3 addressed anxiety/obsessive-compulsive disorder,[18,24,27] and the remaining 2 addressed attention-deficit/hyperactivity disorder (ADHD)[28] and disruptive behavior disorders.[25] None of the included studies were from the same investigators or described the same intervention.

Characterization of the mHealth Interventions

The mHealth interventions studied included 5 different mobile phone apps.[18,22,23,26–28] The remaining 3 studies[18,24,25] all used text messaging and/or multimedia components that were not aggregated into a single app. Hardware and operating systems varied and included mobile phones, tablets,[24,28] and PDAs[26] across Apple, Windows, and Android platforms. Only one study involved wearable technology (an electrodermal sensor).[28] Of the included studies, the Mayo Clinic Anxiety Coach is the only intervention available to the public.[23] All but one of the interventions were explicitly identified as adjunctive tools used to enhance an evidence-based psychotherapeutic intervention: 5 were CBT[18,22–24,26] and 2 were behavioral parent training.[25,28] The exception was a mood journal used in conjunction with a therapist, but the specific therapy was not identified.[27]

Study Characterization and Outcomes

Sample sizes ranged from 2[24] to 855,[18] with most (6) having a sample size of less than 20. Three studies included control groups[18,24,25] and between-group assessments. All studies assessed feasibility at some level, and this was the only outcome assessed for half of the studies. Assessment was done using a combination of direct observation, app usage data, standardized questionnaires, and interviews. Studies that included app usage data[18,22,27] showed typically high user engagement. Questionnaires and interviews yielded generally positive results with most subjects, indicating satisfaction with the interventions.

None of the studies showed that the intervention led to an improvement in clinical outcome because only 3 studies included symptomatic improvement outcomes using standardized rating scales.[23–25] Of these, only 2 were compared with a control group[24,25] and each showed a better response in the intervention arm, but neither reached statistical significance because both were limited by small sample sizes.

DISCUSSION

Findings from this literature review suggest that there is a dearth of research on mHealth interventions specific to childhood mental health, with the salient exception of assistive communication and skill modeling apps for children with autism.

The 8 studies that were yielded by our literature scan shared key attributes in that they all described interventions used to enhance psychotherapy and assessed feasibility of the intervention. The proposed mechanisms by which they would enhance the therapy varied, but generally fitted into a few broad categories: improved patient-clinician communication, improved patient and/or clinician education, improved symptom reporting, improved engagement with material outside of sessions, and improved access to therapy resources.

The studies support the notion that mHealth interventions can be used by children and adolescents, and are readily accepted by them. However, most of the results had limited rigor in study design or interpretation, and even feasibility data that indicate high adherence are difficult to interpret. For example, one study[27] compared adherence percentages across very different time intervals; that is, weighing the usage frequency of a child who used an app for 7 days equally with a child who used it for 326 days. Furthermore, most of the studies did not assess for improvements in clinical outcome. The 2 studies[18,25] that compared clinical outcomes with control groups found better outcomes in the intervention group. However, these results were inconclusive because the difference was not statistically significant, but the studies were likely underpowered.

When considering the use of mHealth interventions in treatment, clinicians should keep in mind that this review did not find any mHealth intervention that has strong evidence of improved clinical outcomes for children with a mental disorder. Although mHealth interventions do not carry the same level of risks and side effects as some other treatments, such as prescription medication, they do carry opportunity costs, including: the purchase cost of the app, the time invested by the clinician in learning the app and by the patient in using it regularly, and potential privacy risks. In addition, the nature of this work is such that studies are frequently authored by those who have helped create the intervention, and the studies present a high risk for positive bias because these investigators often stand to benefit monetarily from the success of the intervention. Two studies declared this as a conflict of interest.[23,24] Clinicians should consider each of these factors when examining new mHealth interventions.

Other Domains Beyond the Scope of this Study

Young adults

By intent, this review excluded interventions studied in young adults (aged 18 years to the early 20s) because the dynamics of mental health care in young adulthood are notably different from those of children less than age 18 years. Although adolescent patients may interact with mobile technology in a fashion similar to young adults, the context of their treatment can be different because they generally remain in the home, under parental authority, and are attending school.

Autism

In addition to the data presented in this article, our initial search revealed that almost all published research on mHealth interventions designed for child mental health treatment focuses on autism spectrum disorders. Most of these interventions are either augmentative and alternative communication devices or some type of skills training and/or modeling program. Our original search included 21 such articles, and a preliminary manual review revealed more than 25 additional articles. The authors chose to exclude articles on this topic because these interventions address different needs from those faced in general child psychiatry, and because this is a specialized area outside the authors' expertise. Instead, interested readers are referred to several previously published reviews.[19–21]

Study Limitations

A potential limitation of this review is that mHealth is still a new field with little consensus on the descriptive terminology such as app versus application.[29] The authors crafted the search algorithm to be as broad as possible, but realize that we may have missed studies using alternative technology that we had not considered, or alternative terms for the same devices (eg, mobile phone vs smartphone, or tablet vs PDA). In addition, some articles with primary investigators from a design/technical background used unconventional or nonclinical terminology to describe clinical interventions; for example, "fear therapy" rather than phobia or anxiety. Furthermore, ambiguity remains about what sorts of interventions should be considered under the umbrella of mHealth. Does the term encompass any type of ecological momentary assessment or only those with certain features?

A second limitation was our choice of 3 citation databases: PubMed and PsycINFO are major databases for medical, behavioral, health, and life science articles, whereas SCOPUS is one of the largest non–domain-specific databases. Although our decision to focus on these 3 databases yielded articles intended for mental health practitioners who would be using such apps, there may be alternative subject-specific databases that could be included to improve the likelihood of finding articles published for a technical audience.

In addition, our decisions to limit the age range to children less than 18 years old and to focus exclusively on studies that use research subjects with a mental health diagnosis and present some form of outcome results has no doubt excluded interventions and apps that are still in the design stage, as well as apps that are not uniquely tailored to children but might be appropriate for child patients. For example, Matthews and colleagues,[30] whose study of the Mobile Mood Diary met our inclusion criteria,[27] had previously published data in a nonclinical sample. Another group has also published several articles about a randomized controlled trial studying a different self-monitoring app, but the study age range was 14 to 24 years.[31,32]

Future Research

Childhood mental health care provides both the opportunity and the necessity of involving people outside the clinician-patient dyad. Several of the studies involved parents to varying degrees and 2 of the apps[25,28] were specifically designed for parent use. However, future interventions may benefit by also including school-based partners, such as counselors or teachers. Children spend a significant amount of time in school and target symptoms may be most prominent at school, such that improved communication between school staff and clinicians may be of great benefit. Although this review found several studies designed to enhance psychotherapy, it did not reveal any that were designed to improve diagnosis or improve pharmacotherapy. Improved data collection from multiple parties could aid clinicians in determining diagnosis and improve consistency with national treatment guidelines that recommend establishing a mechanism for feedback from parents and key informants.[33] mHealth interventions could also potentially aid in improving medication adherence. In addition, disorders that often present differently in early childhood, such as major depression, may require adaptation to overcome obstacles such as lower intelligence and insight in that age group; this may be an area in which passive data collection and physiologic monitoring could yield insight into children who are unable to express their subjective experience.

SUMMARY

MHealth is a promising domain for the development of child mental health interventions because of the increasingly ubiquitous role of mobile technology in the lives of teens and children. Early studies suggest that such interventions are feasible in this population, but more rigorously designed large-scale studies are needed to examine their effectiveness and support their clinical use.

REFERENCES

1. Lenhart A. Teens, social media & technology. Washington, DC: Pew Internet & American Life Project; 2015. Available at: http://www.pewinternet.org/2015/04/09/teens-social-media-technology-2015/. Accessed May 29, 2016.

2. Englander EK. Research Findings: MARC 2011 Survey Grades 3–12. MARC Research Reports. 2011. Available at: http://vc.bridgew.edu/marc_reports/2/. Accessed May 29, 2016.

3. Nielsen LH. SMS Text Messaging Tops Mobile Phone Calling; 2008. Available at: http://www.nielsen.com/us/en/insights/news/2008/in-us-text-messaging-tops-mobile-phone-calling.html. Accessed May 23, 2016.

4. Smith A, Page D. The smartphone difference. Washington, DC: Pew Research Center; 2015. Available at: http://www.pewinternet.org/2015/04/01/us-smartphone-use-in-2015/. Accessed May 29, 2016.

5. Newport F. Most U.S. smartphone owners check phones at least hourly. Washington, DC: Gallup; 2015. Available at: http://www.gallup.com/poll/184046/smartphone-owners-check-phone-least-hourly.aspx. Accessed May 23, 2016.

6. Lenhart A. Cell phone ownership. In: Teens, smartphones & texting. Washington, DC: Pew Research Center; 2012. Available at: http://www.pewinternet.org/2012/03/19/cell-phone-ownership/. Accessed May 29, 2016.

7. Common Sense Media. Zero to eight: children's media use in America 2013. San Francisco (CA): Common Sense Media; 2013. Available at: https://www.commonsensemedia.org/sites/default/files/research/zero-to-eight-2013.pdf. Accessed May 31, 2016.

8. Whittaker R, McRobbie H, Bullen C, et al. Mobile phone-based interventions for smoking cessation. Cochrane Database Syst Rev 2016;(4):CD006611.

9. Liang X, Wang Q, Yang X, et al. Effect of mobile phone intervention for diabetes on glycaemic control: a meta-analysis. Diabet Med 2011;28(4):455–63.

10. Flores Mateo G, Granado-Font E, Ferre-Grau C, et al. Mobile phone apps to promote weight loss and increase physical activity: a systematic review and meta-analysis. J Med Internet Res 2015;17(11):e253.

11. Marcano Belisario JS, Huckvale K, Greenfield G, et al. Smartphone and tablet self management apps for asthma. Cochrane Database Syst Rev 2013;(11):CD010013.

12. Watts S, Mackenzie A, Thomas C, et al. CBT for depression: a pilot RCT comparing mobile phone vs. computer. BMC Psychiatry 2013;13:49.

13. Shapiro JR, Bauer S, Andrews E, et al. Mobile therapy: use of text-messaging in the treatment of bulimia nervosa. Int J Eat Disord 2010;43(6):513–9.

14. Martinez-Perez B, de la Torre-Diez I, Lopez-Coronado M. Mobile health applications for the most prevalent conditions by the World Health Organization: review and analysis. J Med Internet Res 2013;15(6):e120.

15. Huguet A, Rao S, McGrath PJ, et al. A systematic review of cognitive behavioral therapy and behavioral activation apps for depression. PLoS One 2016;11(5):e0154248.

16. Leigh S, Flatt S. App-based psychological interventions: friend or foe? Evid Based Ment Health 2015;18:97–9.

17. Arksey H, O'Malley L. Scoping studies: towards a methodological framework. Int J Soc Res Methodol 2015;8:19–32.

18. Whittaker R, Merry S, Stasiak K, et al. MEMO—A Mobile phone depression prevention intervention for adolescents: development process and postprogram findings on acceptability from a randomized controlled trial. J Med Internet Res 2012;14(1):e13.

19. Schlosser RW, Koul RK. Speech output technologies in interventions for individuals with autism spectrum disorders: a scoping review. Augment Altern Commun 2015;31(14):285–309.

20. Aresti-Bartolome N, Garcia-Zapirain B. Technologies as support tools for persons with autistic spectrum disorder: a systematic review. Int J Environ Res Public Health 2014;11:7767–802.

21. Boyd TK, Barnett JBH, More CM. Evaluating iPad technology for enhancing communication skills of children with autism spectrum disorders. Intervention in School and Clinic 2015;51(1):19–27.

22. Pramana G, Parmanto B, Kendall PC, et al. The SmartCAT: an m-health platform for ecological momentary intervention in child anxiety treatment. Telemed J E Health 2014;20(5):419–27.
23. Whiteside SPH, Ale CM, Vickers D, et al. Case examples of enhancing pediatric OCD treatment with a smartphone application. Clin Case Stud 2014;13(1):80–94.
24. Kobak KA, Mundt JC, Kennard B. Integrating technology into cognitive behavior therapy for adolescent depression: a pilot study. Ann Gen Psychiatry 2015;14:37.
25. Jones DJ, Forehand R, Cuellar J, et al. Technology-enhanced program for child disruptive behavior disorders: development and pilot randomized control trial. J Clin Child Adolesc Psychol 2014;43(1):88–101.
26. De Sa M, Carrico L. Fear therapy for children - a mobile approach. Proceedings of the 2012 ACM SIGCHI Symposium on Engineering Interactive Computing Systems. Denmark, June 25–26, 2012.
27. Matthews M, Doherty G. In the mood: engaging teenagers in psychotherapy using mobile phones. 29th Annual CHI Conference on Human Factors in Computing Systems. Vancouver, May 7–11, 2011.
28. Pina L, Rowan K, Roseway A, et al. In situ cues for ADHD parenting strategies using mobile technology. 8th International Conference on Pervasive Computing Technologies for Healthcare. Oldenburg (Germany), May 20–23, 2014.
29. Lewis TL, Boissaud-Cooke MA, Aungst TD, et al. Consensus on use of the term "app" versus "application" for reporting of mHealth research. J Med Internet Res 2014;16(7):e174.
30. Matthews M, Doherty G, Sharry J, et al. Mobile phone mood charting for adolescents. Br J Guid Counsell 2008;36:113–29.
31. Kauer SD, Reid SC, Crooke AHD, et al. Self-monitoring using mobile phones in the early stages of adolescent depression: randomized controlled trial. J Med Internet Res 2012;14:e67.
32. Reid SC, Kauer SD, Hearps SJC, et al. A mobile phone application for the assessment and management of youth mental health problems in primary care: a randomized controlled trial. BMC Fam Pract 2011;12:131.
33. Pliszka S, AACAP Work Group on Quality Issues. Practice parameter for the assessment and treatment of children and adolescents with attention-deficit/hyperactivity disorder. J Am Acad Child Adolesc Psychiatry 2007;46(7):894–921.

Using Technology to Improve Treatment Outcomes for Children and Adolescents with Eating Disorders

CrossMark

Alison M. Darcy, PhD*, James Lock, MD, PhD

KEYWORDS

- Eating disorders • Technology • Mobile applications • Massive open online courses
- Anorexia nervosa

KEY POINTS

- This article describes the development of 3 technology-based innovations that aim to improve outcomes for children and adolescents with eating disorders (EDs) by directly addressing issues of scale, access, and generating datasets large enough to stimulate treatment development.
- It discusses the use of massive open online courses (MOOCs), an emerging methodology for online learning, and the use of mobile applications for large-scale dissemination.
- The authors present 3 case studies: (1) the modification of a MOOC methodology for psychotherapy training in manualized family-based therapy (FBT) for adolescents with anorexia nervosa, describing the development of the course as well as the ongoing US National Institutes of Health-funded study to evaluate its impact on clinical outcomes; (2) a modified MOOC platform for the delivery of FBT as a guided self-help intervention for parents of children with anorexia nervosa; and (3) the development of mobile applications as a means of delivering data-driven targeted interventional components to individuals who are not in treatment.

INTRODUCTION

Anorexia nervosa (AN) and bulimia nervosa (BN) are serious psychiatric disorders that constitute an important public health problem in terms of prevalence, cost, morbidity, and mortality.[1,2] Approximately 13% of young women will suffer from a diagnosable

Disclosures: Work described in this paper was funded by National Institutes of Health Grants: 5R33MH096779-05; and 4R44MH108221-02. The latter is a grant awarded to Recovery Record Research, Incorporated, a subsidiary of Recovery Record Incorporated. Other than this grant, Dr. J. Lock and Dr. A.M. Darcy have no financial relationship with Recovery Record Incorporated or any other commercial entity relevant to this article to disclose.
Department of Psychiatry and Behavioral Sciences, Stanford School of Medicine, 401 Quarry Road, Stanford, CA 94305, USA
* Corresponding author.
E-mail address: adarcy@stanford.edu

Child Adolesc Psychiatric Clin N Am 26 (2017) 33–42
http://dx.doi.org/10.1016/j.chc.2016.07.010
1056-4993/17/© 2016 Elsevier Inc. All rights reserved.

childpsych.theclinics.com

eating disorder (ED) in their lifetime.[3] It is just beginning to be understood that disordered eating among young men is far more common than previously believed.[4] Individuals with EDs have elevated mortality rates and high medical costs, and often develop physical and psychiatric comorbidities.[2,4,5] Despite the establishment of clinical practice guidelines for effective treatments,[6] dissemination and implementation of evidence-based treatments have progressed slowly, with only a small proportion of affected individuals seeking and receiving treatment.[4,7] Some of the barriers to treatment include insufficient numbers of adequately trained clinicians,[7] shame associated with the illness,[8] geographic constraints, and substantial costs associated with treatment.[9] These reasons, coupled with the relative rarity of the disorders, have meant that the field has been hampered by a lack of data. This has made treatment development especially challenging and slow relative to other disorders. These difficulties can be summarized as problems of scale, access, and innovation inertia caused by a lack of data.

THE CHALLENGE OF SCALABILITY AND ACCESSIBILITY

The current front-line treatment for adolescents is a specific form of family-based treatment (FBT), which leads to full remission in about 50% of patients initially, outperforming individual approaches in the follow-up phase.[10] Largely a behavioral treatment, it features interventions highly specific to the illness, such as framing progress around weight gain, orchestrating an intense scene around the illness, and a family meal that includes in vivo parental coaching. Given the specificities of the treatment model, specialist training is a necessity. However, training to the level of certification consists of attending a 2-day intensive seminar, with few following up with the required individualized session-by-session supervision on treatment with at least 3 families. Even where this training has been undertaken at an institutional level, the model has not been implemented with fidelity.[10] This inherent lack of scalability is a huge challenge for treatment providers and health systems at a global level.

The net result of these challenges means that most adolescent patients with a diagnosis of AN do not have access to the treatment that is most likely to bring about full and sustained recovery. Thus, the same challenges seen from the point of view of those who have received a diagnosis is a problem of access. The existing disparity between need and availability of specialized treatment for AN is especially alarming given the vital importance of early intervention for maximizing chances of recovery, and the substantial medical and psychosocial consequences if AN persists. Thus, there is an immediate need to invest resources in adapting FBT to be scalable from the perspective of treatment providers and accessible from the perspective of those who need it.

PROBLEMS OF A LACK OF DATA

Although EDs have seen an increase in research interest in recent years, most clinical studies are of adult populations. There are only 7 published randomized clinical trials examining adolescents with AN, totaling just 480 subjects. In BN, few treatments exist that were specifically designed for child and adolescent populations, and extrapolating from treatments of choice for adults (eg, cognitive behavioral therapy) has not proven particularly fruitful, although there are 3 randomized clinical trials examining this population. In AN, there are substantial difficulties associated with conducting research, and among the greatest challenges are the relative rarity of this disorder, and either the resultant lack of statistical power necessary to detect changes, or the time it takes to build adequately powered sample sizes. In a recent review of evidence-based treatments for AN,[11] the authors concluded that relatively little innovation has occurred in the past 80 years. Clearly, more data are needed from which to develop treatments that are customized and specifically address the needs of young people.

OPPORTUNITIES IN TECHNOLOGY TO ADDRESS THESE PROBLEMS

The authors developed 3 innovations to address scalability, lack of access, and data-informed treatment innovation. To address these challenges, they turned to concurrent innovations in the field of online education, in the form of massive open online course (MOOC) platforms. In the field of education, MOOCs have successfully delivered specialist top-tier expertise all over the world in a way that is scalable, solves problems of access, and generates data sets sufficient to stimulate genuine innovation in teaching practices. It was the authors' contention that both these online learning methodologies and the technical platforms on which they were delivered could be leveraged for the purposes of clinical training and the delivery of treatment. Finally, the authors turned to advances in mobile technology, and in particular, smartphones, to first augment, and later deliver, interventions to individuals with EDs who are and are not in formal treatment, respectively.

MASSIVE OPEN ONLINE COURSES

MOOCs represent an emerging methodology in online learning. Some of the defining features of MOOCs that distinguish them from other online learning platforms include that they

1. Rely heavily on video with most material being delivered that way
2. Include a range of assessments that encourage procedural (rather than only declarative or rote) learning
3. Can be data-driven and iteratively enhanced

Some MOOC platforms have leveraged social technology to provide meaningful opportunities for students to collaborate and communicate within a community of learners. These features were leveraged to construct a learning environment ideal for clinical training. One of the defining features of MOOCs that was not used in this case, however, is that they have open, public enrollment.

DEVELOPMENT OF A MASSIVE OPEN ONLINE COURSE-BASED SPECIALIST PSYCHOTHERAPY TRAINING IN FAMILY-BASED THERAPY
The Clinical Training Massive Open Online Course

An online course for FBT was developed on an MOOC platform as part of a US National Institutes of Health (NIH)-funded study to explore the feasibility of improving fidelity to FBT by improving training.

Training was amended to include training modules that specifically target elements of treatment fidelity that influence outcomes. The 12-week course consists of about 6 to 7 lectures, comprising 5 to 6 very short (about 3–4 minutes in length) didactic videos that discuss the treatment model and an accompanying role-play therapy session (or series of short role-played scenarios) with a typical case of AN, prescribed reading, and an assignment. The course is delivered sequentially, with assignments due on Sunday evening and a new lecture delivered every Monday morning. The authors borrowed from concepts of case method teaching[12] to include the kind of clinical information that one would have with a typical AN case (ie, weight chart [with every lecture to track progress], standardized assessments, and intake evaluation report) to create an immersive clinical experience. Assignments tested clinical decision making: "read this intake evaluation and write down which lab and medical tests you would order for this patient given her history," and provided the opportunity to step into the shoes of the experts and rate how well the therapist executes a clinician intervention in a segment of video of role-played therapeutic session.

Pilot Data

The course was not open or public; participants could only enroll by invitation.

In a 6-month period, the authors conducted 3 pilot studies with N = 45 participants, a mix of MD psychiatrists (37%), doctoral-level psychologists (30%), master's level family therapists (7%), doctoral-level graduate students (22%), and 1 registered dietician (4%). Completion (defined as finishing >80% of videos and assignments) ranged from 40% in the first pilot to 78% in the final. There was a high level of satisfaction with the course overall (85%), the didactic content (100%), the clinical content including role-play videos, and supportive clinical material (80%) and the homework (69%). Not having enough time was the most frequently cited challenge to completing the course (70%). This was also demonstrated by the fact that 76% of participants completed their course obligations on the weekend after 8 PM. Ninety-four percent of participants said they were satisfied with the usability of the interface. Development of the training model was iterative, with feedback being integrated into the next pilot iteration. For example, participants in the first pilot strongly suggested implementing more structure around homework assignments (eg, being due on a consistent day of the week for each lecture, frequent email reminders), and so this was adjusted in the second pilot. In the second iteration, participants suggested more opportunity for discussion of actual clinical cases, and a thus a system of moderated asynchronous clinical discussion was implemented in the third pilot. This system of iterative development led to more innovation in training methods than has been possible in the previous decade of traditional seminar-based training.

Next Steps

For the randomized trial, and unlike most studies of online training interventions, the authors will measure clinical outcomes and benchmark against known outcomes from previous trials where standard training has been implemented. They are developing 2 methods of assessing applied knowledge acquisition and clinical skill. Applied knowledge is tested by a written, clinical vignette, and multiple choice -examination, and to measure clinical skill, trainees are required to respond to a series of short, standardized role-played video vignettes as if they were the therapist. The teleconference recordings are then expert-rated using a validated measure of treatment fidelity.[10]

DEVELOPMENT OF INTERNET-DELIVERED GUIDED SELF-HELP
Background

Internet-delivered interventions present the opportunity to increase access, reach, reduce costs, and establish sustainable systems for providing care. When linked to in-person medical services, such as monitoring by a pediatrician, online programs may help reduce mental health care disparities for adolescent AN. Internet-delivered guided self-help (GSH) interventions have been successfully implemented among individuals with BN and binge eating disorder, and at a minimum appear to promote symptom reduction beyond a wait list control condition.[13–16] There are currently no comparable treatments developed for AN. A fundamental principle of FBT is parental empowerment, making it ideal for dissemination as a GSH approach for parents. The authors' research team developed an Internet-delivered GSH parent intervention derived from FBT for the prevention of AN and early intervention. Pilot data suggested that an Internet-delivered text-based program was feasible to provide, acceptable to parents, and may result in symptom reduction in both those who are at risk of developing AN and those with an ED not otherwise specified.[17] A natural and important extension of this preliminary work was the examination of its utility for parents of adolescents with full AN. The authors ran a case series to answer the question of whether FBT could be adapted and delivered as an online GSH intervention for parents of adolescents with AN. Data gathered in the case series will be benchmarked against a large body of existing data from trials that have examined traditional FBT to gather preliminary information on the efficacy of a GSH approach to FBT (FBT-GSH).

The Intervention

The program consisted of 80 short videos (all <7 minutes in length, average length about 3 minutes) delivered in 10 lectures over 6 months. Incorporating a participatory medicine framework, the authors included 3 25-minute videos featuring an interview with a recovery role model, a former patient successfully treated with FBT for AN. In addition to the videos, materials aimed at empowering parents in the active treatment of their adolescents were uploaded. These included materials that are commonly used clinically such as an ideal body weight calculator (using growth charts as reference tables), a weight chart to allow parents to plot weight progress, and a booklet explaining medical management of AN (produced by the Academy of Eating Disorders). A recipe book produced by parents who have experience of renourishment was also uploaded, and each family was sent a copy of the self-help book "Help Your Teenager Beat an Eating Disorder," 2nd Edition (Lock & Le Grange, 2014) from which readings were prescribed weekly. Finally, the therapist conducted brief (30-min) check-in meetings with parents over a Heath Insurance Portability and Accountability Act (HIPAA)-compliant video conferencing program. Following the form factor of gold-standard FBT, these meetings were initially weekly, but tapered off to every 2 to 3 weeks during later phases of treatment and finally at monthly intervals for the final sessions. All families had exactly 12 check-in sessions with a certified FBT practitioner.

Rather than provide in vivo coaching as in standard FBT, the assessment capability of the MOOC platform was leveraged to create opportunities for parents to develop skills needed for successfully navigating the renourishment process. In this way, parents were encouraged to adopt an objective observational orientation (**Fig. 1**), and the data gathered were discussed during the weekly check-in with the therapist.

To ensure that there was no delay before getting treatment, a rolling group format was implemented such that individuals could join the group as soon as they were eligible.

As described previously, the MOOC platform contains a discussion forum that aims to facilitate the establishment of learning communities. In the context of the GSH program, the forum became an asynchronous support group addressing the sense of isolation that parents often report feeling.

Pilot Data

A small case series is currently underway to test the feasibility and acceptability of the intervention. The overall study design was a case series of 20 parents of adolescents (aged 11–18 years) with a diagnosis of AN in the previous 12 months. To allow for benchmarking against data that have been collected from randomized clinical trials at Stanford and University of Chicago, the authors maintained the same inclusion

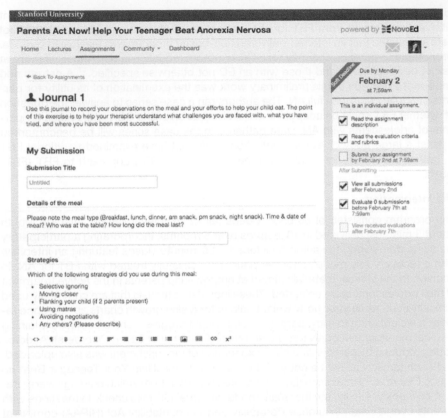

Fig. 1. The authors' research team developed an Internet-delivered GSH parent intervention for the treatment of AN translating therapeutic coaching into meaningful assignments. (*Courtesy of* Stanford University, Stanford, CA; with permission.)

criteria of weight between 75% to 90% of expected for age and height. Prior to enrollment, all participants must get sign-off from a treating physician to certify that the patient is safe for outpatient therapy and to continue medical monitoring. At the time of writing, 16 families have completed treatment, and while outcomes have not been formally evaluated, there are interim findings for the first 11 families who completed. The parents of N = 20 adolescents were recruited (mean age = 14.8; standard deviation [SD] = 1.9) with a mean % expected body weight (for age and height) of 83% (SD = 5.27%).

Although follow-up data are not available at this time, among the 11 participants who have completed the program, there was a significant reduction in symptoms between baseline and end of treatment. Percent expected body weight for age and height (EBW) increased from a mean of 82.37% (SD = 5.96) at baseline to 97.23% by end of treatment (SD = 7.98) with a large effect size (Cohen d = 1.94). The restraint subscale of the Eating Disorders Examination Questionnaire decreased significantly (with a large effect size of .71).

Again, while only in a position to report interim findings, data suggest that outcomes from this study are within the range of those achieved by comparison FBT trials. For example, the effect size of 1.94 compares favorably to the within subjects change in weight among a pooled dataset of N = 196 adolescents treated during comparison FBT trials that demonstrated a significant weight increase between baseline and end of treatment with a large effect size of 1.2. In addition, 60% of the adolescents met criteria for full remission at end of treatment (defined as weight at least 95% of expected and Eating Disorders Examination Questionnaire global score within 1 SD of published norms). This compares favorably to a rate of about 42% in the Lock and colleagues[18] study and 33% in the Agras and colleagues[19] study.

Although these findings are interim, the authors are optimistic about the success of the study overall. The study appears to be feasible and acceptable to parents, and patient safety considerations appear to be appropriate.

DEVELOPING SMARTPHONE APPLICATIONS FOR THE AUGMENTATION AND DELIVERY OF THERAPEUTIC INTERVENTIONS
Background

Smart mobile technologies offer unique opportunity to dramatically change the landscape of therapeutic intervention. However, as is the case across almost all diagnoses, the amount of available smartphone applications claiming to impart some kind of mental health advantage for their users far outweighs the evidence that confirms such assertions. The first studies on mobile-enhanced therapeutic interventions in EDs, although limited, were promising, although most pertained to short messaging system (SMS) interventions, or ecological momentary assessment. However, 2 reports demonstrated increased adherence to smartphone self-monitoring over paper and pen for recording meals[20] and physical activity.[21]

Food for Thought

The authors first developed a Web application optimized for smartphone called Food For Thought.[22] Developed in the context of a treatment trial for adolescent BN, they created an application in the hope that it would facilitate adolescents' food and symptom self-monitoring. The application was built using an academic development approach, emulating as close as possible the conventional paper-and-pen format and with great attention paid to encryption and secure hosting. The latter piece necessitated substantial time investment before the application was ready for roll-out with patients but had the advantage of ensuring patient confidentiality. The authors ran a small case series of the first 5 users of the applications and their respective clinicians, demonstrating feasibility and acceptability as well as broad heterogeneity in terms of how it was used.[22] Building an application for research purposes had the advantages of being HIPAA-compliant; however, without a dedicated team to support and update the application, it quickly became outdated.

The Development of Recovery Record

Around the same time, the authors began consulting with an entrepreneur who wanted to build a mobile application to enhance treatment for EDs and facilitate food and symptom self-monitoring. This application was developed using best-practice in person-centered design, soliciting user feedback in rapid, iterative development cycles and implementing current understanding in user engagement. The development process is described in detail elsewhere.[23] The result is a mature and highly acceptable application that has been downloaded by over 300,000 individuals. Although this reach may be modest for most large-scale commercial applications, this kind of reach for an ED service is unprecedented, and, outside the context of only the best-executed and large-scale epidemiologic studies, the dataset it generates is unique.

Most users are young, with the mean reported age being 22 (range = 13–77 years) and about two-thirds of those who provide their age being under the age of 25.

Using Mobile Data to Develop Targeted Treatment for Individuals Not in Formal Treatment

Although the application was originally developed to facilitate evidence-based treatment, preliminary analyses suggested that approximately 46% of application users were not currently in therapy. In addition, approximately 26% of these individuals saw clinically significant symptom improvement after at least 4 weeks of application usage. This overall response rate is comparable to those observed in clinical trials of self-help interventions, although these are not directly comparable. However, a limitation of the application is that it is a "one-size-fits-all" product that does not formally account for the heterogeneity of ED symptoms. Genetic, personality, and neurocognitive data support distinct clusters of ED presentations that also differ according to response to treatment and course, and the authors' preliminary data strongly suggested that Recovery Record users span the breadth of this spectrum, offering a unique opportunity to specifically engage diagnostic verticals from 1 platform.

Next Steps

In partnership with Recovery Record, the authors obtained a 2-phase Small Business Innovation Grant from NIH to capitalize on this public health opportunity and develop content tailored to the needs of specific user groups according to their symptoms.

The study is nearing completion of its first phase, the aim of which is to confirm the algorithms that were generated by analysis of the first dataset in a prospective design to minimize bias. To date, the authors have recruited N = 1276 individuals and have developed curated content that addresses their symptoms. The authors have completed a patient-centered design process to create content and curated it into 5 distinct programs that incorporate review and feedback on the previous week's progress gathered on the application, goal setting and skills selection, as well as activities that facilitate psychoeducation. Although they have consulted with service users throughout the process, initial pilot data suggest feasibility and acceptability of the programs. In the randomized controlled trial phase of the project, the authors will test whether the resultant algorithm-generated dynamic programs delivered in an adaptive application will improve outcomes relative to the standard "one-size-fits-all" version.

This methodology represents a data-driven approach to service development for individuals with EDs. There are several reasons to believe that if successful, Recovery Record has the potential to make a substantial public health impact. As the first commercially available smartphone application developed specifically for EDs crossing ages and diagnostic boundaries, it represents an important opportunity for reaching a population that is notoriously difficult to reach. In addition, the incremental cost of delivering tailored intervention components is negligible in comparison to traditional interventions, especially if reach is taken into consideration.

SUMMARY

The authors' research group at Stanford has sought to tackle the many barriers that face adolescents with EDs and evidence-based service providers with a view to improving clinical outcomes and prevention efforts. In doing so, they have learned that the most successful strategies come from looking outward from one's psychiatric subspecialty, toward parallel innovations and complementary expertise. The authors advocate for the development of fruitful partnerships with computer scientists and companies with deep domain expertise in specific technology verticals, as these result in mutually beneficial relationships and the development of services that reflect best practices in both technology and clinical service design. From both perspectives, an emphasis on patient-centered (/human-centered) design practice should be adopted to ensure ethics in clinical design thinking at every stage of development.

REFERENCES

1. Stice E, Marti CN, Rohde P. Prevalence, incidence, impairment, and course of the proposed DSM-5 eating disorder diagnoses in an 8-year prospective community study of young women. Int J Eat Disord 2013;122:445–57.
2. Stuhldreher N, Konnopka A, Wild B, et al. Cost-of-illness studies and cost-effectiveness analyses in eating disorders: a systematic review. Int J Eat Disord 2012;45(4):476–91.
3. Swanson S, Scott J, Crow Le Grange D, et al. Prevalence and correlates of eating disorders in adolescents. Results from the national comorbidity survey replication adolescent supplement. Arch Gen Psychiatry 2011;68:714–23.
4. Hoek HW. Incidence, prevalence and mortality of anorexia nervosa and other eating disorders. Curr Opin Psychiatry 2006;19(4):389–94.
5. Agras WS. The consequences and costs of the eating disorders. Psychiatr Clin North Am 2001;24(2):371–9.
6. Wilson GT, Fairburn CG. Treatments for eating disorders. In: Nathan PE, Gorman JM, editors. Treatments that work. New York: Oxford University Press; 1998. p. 501–3.
7. Hart LM, Granillo M, Jorm AF, et al. Unmet need for treatment in the eating disorders: a systematic review of eating disorder specific treatment seeking among community cases. Clin Psychol Rev 2011;31(5):727–35.
8. Fairburn CG, Hay PJ, Welch SL. Binge eating and bulimia nervosa: distribution and determinants. In: Fairburn CG, Wilson GT, editors. Binge eating: nature, assessment, and treatment. New York: Guilford Press; 1993. p. 123–43.
9. Burns JM, Durkin L, Nicholas J. Mental health of young people in the United States: what role can the Internet play in reducing stigma and promoting help-seeking? J Adolesc Health 2009;45:95–7.
10. Forsberg S, Fitzpatrick KK, Darcy A, et al. Development and evaluation of a treatment fidelity instrument for family-based treatment of adolescent anorexia nervosa. Int J Eat Disord 2015;48(1):91–9.
11. Fairburn G, Patel V. The global dissemination of psychological treatments: a roadmap for research and practice. Am J Psychiatry 2014;171:495–8.
12. Austin SB, Sonneville KR. Closing the "know-do" gap: training public health professionals in eating disorders prevention via case-method teaching. Int J Eat Disord 2013;46(5):533–7.
13. Carrard I, Crepin C, Rouget P, et al. Randomised controlled trial of a guided self-help treatment on the Internet for binge eating disorder. Behav Res Ther 2011; 49(8):482–91.
14. Jones M, Luce KH, Osborne MI, et al. Randomized, controlled trial of an internet-facilitated intervention for reducing binge eating and overweight in adolescents. Pediatrics 2008;121(3):453–62.
15. Ljotsson B, Lundin C, Mitsell K, et al. Remote treatment of bulimia nervosa and binge eating disorder: a randomized trial of Internet-assisted cognitive behavioural therapy. Behav Res Ther 2007;45(4):649–61.

16. Sánchez-Ortiz VC, Munro C, Stahl D, et al. A randomized controlled trial of internet-based cognitive-behavioural therapy for bulimia nervosa or related disorders in a student population. Psychol Med 2011;41(2):407–17.
17. Jones M, Volker U, Lock J, et al. Family-based early intervention for anorexia nervosa. Eur Eat Disord Rev 2012;20(3):e137–43.
18. Lock J, Le Grange D, Agras WS, et al. Randomized clinical trial comparing family-based treatment with adolescent-focused individual therapy for adolescents with anorexia nervosa. Arch Gen Psychiatry 2010;67(10):1025–32.
19. Agras WS, Lock J, Brandt H, et al. Comparison of 2 family therapies for adolescent anorexia nervosa: a randomized parallel trial. JAMA Psychiatry 2014;71(11): 1279–86.
20. Carter MC, Burley VJ, Nykjaer C, et al. Adherence to a smartphone application for weight loss compared to website and paper diary: pilot randomized controlled trial. J Med Internet Res 2013;15(4):e32.
21. Kirwan M, Duncan MJ, Vandelanotte C, et al. Using smartphone technology to monitor physical activity in the 10,000 Steps program: a matched case–control trial. J Med Internet Res 2012;14(2):e55.
22. Darcy AM, Adler S, Miner A, et al. How smartphone applications may be implemented in the treatment of eating disorders: case reports and case series data. Adv Eat Disor: Theory, Research and Practice 2014;2(3):217–32.
23. Tregarthen JP, Lock J, Darcy AM. Development of a smartphone application for eating disorder self-monitoring. Int J Eat Disord 2015;48(7):972–82.

Patient Portals in Child and Adolescent Psychiatry

Ernest Jeremy Kendrick, MD[a],*, Christy Benson, BA[b]

KEYWORDS

- Patient portals • Child and adolescent psychiatry • Confidentiality
- Health information technology • Personal health record

KEY POINTS

- Patient portals are secure Web sites that give patients access to personal health information and the ability to securely communicate with their providers.
- While little data exist about their use in child and adolescent psychiatry, patient portals present a unique opportunity to interact with young patients.
- Important issues regarding confidentiality must be considered when adopting a patient portal for the child/adolescent population.
- With attention to local, state, and federal regulations, access policies can be created that help mitigate concerns about confidentiality with patient portals.

INTRODUCTION

The rise of health information technology has led to significant changes in the way physicians practice medicine and interact with their patients. Volumes of easily accessed medical information through the Internet have led to a shift in autonomy and engagement for patients in their own health care. One area of health information technology that has facilitated this empowerment is the use of patient portals. Portals offer patients the opportunity to more closely interface with their own health care in a variety of ways. Themes of autonomy and independence are hallmarks of development for children and adolescents. Therefore, ensuring these young patients have meaningful and productive access to patient portals is important. The purpose of this article is to describe and explore the use of patient portals in child and adolescent psychiatry.

HealthIT.gov describes a patient portal as "a secure online website that gives patients convenient 24-hour access to personal health information from anywhere with an Internet connection."[1] Portals have developed alongside electronic health records systems with

Disclosures: The authors have nothing to disclose.
[a] Department of Psychiatry, University of Utah School of Medicine, 501 Chipeta Way, Salt Lake City, UT 84108, USA; [b] Information Technology Services, University of Utah, 585 Komas Drive, Salt Lake City, UT 84108, USA
* Corresponding author.
E-mail address: jeremy.kendrick@hsc.utah.edu

Child Adolesc Psychiatric Clin N Am 26 (2017) 43–54
http://dx.doi.org/10.1016/j.chc.2016.07.005
1056-4993/17/© 2016 Elsevier Inc. All rights reserved.
childpsych.theclinics.com

the belief that the systems will enhance patient satisfaction and improve care.[2] Portals offer patients an interface by which they can explore and understand details of their health.

Patient portals accessed by child and adolescent patients provide a unique opportunity and challenge for health care providers to more closely work with this unique population. Not surprisingly, the body of literature exploring the utilization and complexity of child and adolescent health care portals is small.[2] The majority of literature that does exist is limited mostly to adolescent medicine and to pediatric medical practices for patients with chronic health care needs. There is little to no information available in the literature giving specific attention to portals in child and adolescent psychiatry. A PubMed search performed in April 2016 using the parameters "('Patient portal' [All Fields] AND ('adolescent psychiatry' [MeSH Terms] OR 'child psychiatry' [MeSH Terms]))" shows no studies to date.

This article provides a brief summary of the definition and potential scope of child and adolescent patient portals, and briefly reviews the literature that does exist in adolescent medicine with an eye to how this information might apply to child and adolescent psychiatry. The article covers technical aspects regarding the implementation and policy surrounding portals for child and adolescent patients as part of an enterprise EMR (electronic medical record) and ends with a discussion of the challenges and potential solutions for patient portals.

PATIENT PORTALS: GENERAL PRINCIPLES

A broad discussion (age- and specialty-independent) of patient portals is a helpful starting place for learning about their use and implementation.

Although patient portals have been around since the late 1990s, the inclusion of patient engagement measures in the US Centers for Medicare and Medicaid Services' meaningful use incentive program have pushed portals into a position of prominence over the last 5 years. This has meant more IT (information technology) vendors entering the market with portal solutions, better technology offerings in these portals, more providers offering portal solutions to their patients, and more patients accessing their health information through portals. Portals associated with a provider's EMR enjoy greater market share over portal solutions that can only offer patients a repository to collect their own health information.[3]

There is no standard set of features that must be included in a portal; however, the meaningful use requirements have helped to canonize certain features. Meaningful Use Measure: Objective 8, titled Patient Electronic Access, requires that patients are provided with timely electronic access to their health information, including laboratory results, problem lists, medication lists, and allergies. This means most of today's portals allow patients to view these items from their EMR. Objective 9 for eligible providers, Secure Messaging, sets requirements around using secure electronic messaging to communicate with patients on relevant health information.[4] This has driven successful patient portals to include mechanisms for secure messaging between patients and providers.

Table 1 outlines common clinical portal features, showing view-only information versus interactive features.

It is also common for portals to provide access to health systems' data that are not necessarily clinical in nature. This can include bills, insurance benefits and claims, and appointment scheduling. Although these features can provide value and convenience for patients, this article focuses on the clinical aspects of patient portals.

Mining portal usage data at the University of Utah Healthcare System one can easily identify that secure messaging is the most popular features with patients (**Table 2**).

Table 1
Common clinical patient portal features

Information Patients Can Access (View Only)	Opportunities for Patient/Provider Interaction
• Lab results • Summaries of outpatient doctor visits • Hospital discharge summaries • Medications and prescription details • Immunization histories • Problem (diagnosis) list • Allergies • Health education materials	• Exchange secure E-mail with their health care teams • Complete forms and questionnaires • Request prescription refills • Record and share home health monitoring information (eg, blood pressure, blood glucose, weight, and medication adherence) • E-visits • Preventive care reminders that prompt patients to schedule routine screenings or vaccinations

The University of Utah Healthcare System launched its patient portal in 2010 and currently has over 190,000 patients with a portal account. Looking at the most recent monthly data from 2016, almost 60% of patients who logged into the portal accessed the messaging feature.

With some understanding of what types of options are available in patient portals, it becomes important to understand and address the differences in how these features work for children and adolescents. Although much of the same information is available for adults and child/adolescent patients, details of what, how, and with whom that information is shared becomes important.

POTENTIAL SENSITIVE TOPICS IN PATIENT PORTALS

Although the practice of adolescent medicine across a number of specialties presents an opportunity for potentially sensitive information to be shared and disclosed, child and adolescent psychiatry generally is unique in the amount and depth to which these

Table 2
University of Utah Health Care: top 10 clinical features in the patient portal

Rank	Feature	Count of Unique Users Who Accessed the Feature	Percent of Total Unique Users Who Accessed the Feature
1	Secure messaging	28,342	59.79%
2	Laboratory test results	20,109	42.42%
3	Preventive care	17,685	37.31%
4	Upcoming appointment details	12,715	26.82%
5	Medications	11,324	23.89%
6	Problem list	9,803	20.68%
7	Allergies	9,741	20.55%
8	Immunizations	9,386	19.80%
9	Outpatient visit summary	7,042	14.86%
10	Letters—view list or details	5,684	11.99%

Patient access occurring from 4/1/2016 through 4/30/2016.
Total unique users who accessed the portal: 47,400.

topics are explored. Specific areas of concern have been identified in the literature, and patient portal systems should pay particular attention to these topics and securing access to them appropriately (**Table 3**).

Protecting young patients from breaches of confidentiality in these areas is difficult. It requires vigilant monitoring of what information is disclosed and significant planning and thoughtful implementation of a portal system serving child and adolescent patients.

DOCUMENTATION IN PATIENT PORTALS

One area in which patient portals are extending unfiltered access to health information for patients is through ready access to provider documentation. Although patients have always had access to their medical record through formal requests, this process has often been burdensome and time consuming. Allowing patients to access the documentation related to their visits through patient portals offers this information without the hurdles and pitfalls of classic medical record requests. OpenNotes is an initiative that advocates for access to clinical documentation by patients through the patient portal.[5] The OpenNotes Web site estimates that more than 7 million patients have access to clinicians' notes through the initiative, with access being granted at more than 50 large medical systems, including the Veterans Affairs (VA) system.[6] There have not been any documented trials of OpenNotes specific to pediatric populations. Further research and a thoughtful approach to the implications of open documentation in this population are needed.

Table 3
Specific areas of concern to be protected against breaches of confidentiality

Sensitive Topics	Problem list	Medication list	Lab Results	Documentation	Billing	Scheduling
			Area in Portal for Potential Breach in Confidentiality			
Details regarding family planning/ sexual activity	X	X	X	X	X	X
Sexually transmitted infections	X	X	X	X	X	X
Substance abuse	X	X	X	X	X	X
Sexual orientation				X		
Gender identity	X	X	X	X	X	X
Sensitive psychosocial details (eg, parental preference or friendships)	X		X	X	X	X
Results/presence of psychological testing	X			X	X	X

There are data in the OpenNotes literature showing that patients appreciate and want access to this information. Although concerns about privacy exist, many patients agree that access to this information is helpful.[7]

Data describing the implementation, utilization, and outcomes of extending access to documentation in the child and adolescent mental health population are sparse. There are survey data of mental health providers; however, those data are limited to adult practitioners. One study of mental health providers in the VA system showed that although most generally think the concept of open documentation is a good idea, only 50% supported extending this transparency to mental health documentation. Most clinicians studied reported significant changes in the level of detail and tone of their documentation secondary to concerns that patients will have easy access to the information.[8]

The authors' own health system at the University of Utah planned to role out Open-Notes in mid-2016. The concerns of some mental health clinicians shown in the literature are echoed in the University of Utah system's approach to initially withhold mental health documentation from the first year of OpenNotes rollout. More data and information are needed to truly judge clinician and patient preference in regards to accessing mental health documentation, especially in the child and adolescent population.

APPROACHES TO STRUCTURING ACCESS IN CHILD/ADOLESCENT PORTALS

Given the large amount of data available in the medical record and potentially accessible through patient portals, significant thought must be given to who is granted access to any particular part of the portal and its corresponding sensitive data. This is generally accomplished through developing access policies that implement security and establish limits to access of certain information based on who is trying to access it.

With the complexity and variability of family structures, portal access policies need to be flexible enough to accommodate any number of guardianship/parental situations. Contentious divorces, changes in guardianship with state involvement, and other custody arrangements present overwhelming complexity in regards to the sharing of medical information of a child or adolescent patient. Mental health records in particular present a uniquely sensitive body of information. Such documentation may contain information that 1 guardian may not want another guardian to know. Sometimes protective orders exist between guardians, and making information available through a patient portal system presents a liability for patients, parents, and/or providers.

There are technological limitations to the identification and withholding of potentially sensitive information. Issues of particular sensitivity to patients in child and adolescent psychiatry may be discussed or identifiable through documentation, laboratory results, problem lists, or billing details, all of which are often areas potentially available through patient portals. With each additional area of the medical record that is opened to access by patients, the risk of breaching confidentiality grows. This again underscores the need for broadly accepted policies and procedures regarding access to the patient portal for patients and their parents.

There are several different models described in the literature that define potential security policies structuring access to health information of minors.[9–11] These different models reflect the differences of opinion between parents and adolescents regarding access to health information. It is up to individual institutions, providers, and local laws and regulations to determine which model best fits the needs of respective institutions.

Most access policy models focus on the period of adolescence. There is fairly common acceptance of access uniformly granted to parents for younger children, and exclusive access for adults after the transition from adolescence. Although local law and policy differs, the age of adolescence generally ranges from a start age of 11 to 14 to the transition to adulthood at age 18.

Models addressing this complicated timeframe of adolescence generally fall into 3 categories. The confidentiality model supports parents relinquishing any access to portal information, with adolescents retaining full access. The family engagement model aims to strike a balance, with parents and teens sharing access, with the understanding that any confidential information accessible through the portal is open to the parents' view in addition to the adolescent's view. The parent orientation model supports full parental oversight, with the adolescent having no unique access to patient portal data.

There are risks and benefits to each model, as summarized in **Table 4**.

The institution of these policies is further complicated by other aspects of the EMR. Access to information available to patients through patient portals has implications as it relates to initiatives for shared access across EMR systems and institutions, as well as the evolving concept of personal controlled health records.[2] Both of these concepts present a complex need to juggle adolescent and parent preference regarding access and policies that may differ across different institutions.[9]

REGULATORY VARIABILITY

In practice, parent and adolescent preferences are often subjugated to concerns over sharing information in violation of HIPAA (Health Insurance Portability and

Table 4
Risks and benefits to the confidentiality model, the family engagement model, and the parent orientation model

	Description	Pros	Cons
Confidentiality	• Parent relinquishes access while adolescent maintains full ownership of portal	• Supports development of autonomy in adolescent patients • Maximizes confidentiality for adolescent patient	• Parental concerns about feeling out of the loop
Family engagement	• Shared access between parents and adolescents.	• Supports discussion and communication between parent and teen • Keeps adolescent engaged in his or her own health with parental oversight	• Not appropriate for sensitive issues inherent to adolescent mental health
Parent orientation	• Parent has full access to adolescent health data. The patient has no unique access.	• Parents retain full control • Minimizes risk of irresponsible use of medical information by adolescent	• Not appropriate for sensitive issues inherent to adolescent mental health • Does not support development of autonomy for adolescent patients

Adapted from Thompson LA, Martinko T, Budd P, et al. Meaningful use of a confidential adolescent patient portal. J Adolesc Health 2016;58(2):136; with permission.

Accountability Act) or state-level privacy laws. The HIPAA privacy rule allows that parents can act as a minor child's personal representative, and in that role, they have full access to the child's medical record. However, HIPAA allows for several exceptions:

1. When the minor is the person who consents to care, and the consent of the parent is not required under state or other applicable law
2. When the minor obtains care at the direction of a court or a person appointed by the court
3. When, and to the extent that the parent agrees that the minor and the health care provider may have a confidential relationship[12]

Complying with these statutes can be challenging for health care institutions. Before releasing information to a parent, providers must monitor for circumstances, court orders, or parenting plans that would prohibit a guardian or parent from having access to the child's medical record.[11]

This first exception, with its deference to state law, makes it impossible to set a national standard for parental access to patient portals. Consent laws for minors do not exist in every state, but where they do, mental health services are frequently set apart as a treatment for which minors can request access. A 2009 report on state medical record access laws found that the age at which a person may lawfully consent to care varies, not just from 1 state to another, but often varies with the health condition at issue. For example, in 1 state, the age of consent is 12 years for treatment of a sexually transmitted disease (STD) and 14 years for treatment of substance abuse."[13] When the report looked specifically for state statutes around outpatient mental health treatment, "twenty-eight states have statutes and/or regulations that expressly permit minors to consent to outpatient mental health treatment." This obviously limits exclusive access to patient portals for adolescents in these cases.

Managing these consents with respect to patient age, applicable service, and the validity of a particular parent–child relationship is a daunting task that is not readily supported by available portal technology. When choosing a patient portal solution, institutions most often select the portal associated with their EMR, as it provides the easiest integration.[3] These EMR-aligned portals create a seamless flow of information between the patient and his or her health care organization, but they often lack the ability to segregate information in a way that can be selectively withheld from the portal. If a parent is given portal access to the adolescent's chart, there may not be a practical mechanism to withhold protected data related to care given under the minor's sole consent.

Because the applicable laws and statutes do not mandate electronic access to medical record information for the parent or the adolescent, many institutions withhold portal access altogether. Parents are commonly given full portal access for young children, but at the age of adolescence, that access is terminated. This is most common in states where law allows adolescents to consent to treatment for particular services like mental health, but this practice can be found in other states too.

When there is no state law prohibiting parental access to a minor's chart, HIPAA allows the licensed health care provider to exercise his or her professional judgment to grant or deny parental access to the minor's medical information.[12] If the EMR and portal solution does not provide a mechanism for withholding information on sensitive topics, organizations may choose to err on the side of caution and revoke portal access altogether.

As meaningful use and its evolution into the future Medicare Access and CHIP Reauthorization Act regulatory programs continue to push the envelope of patient engagement, eligible providers and hospitals are pushing technology vendors to offer better solutions. Pediatric organizations, in particular, cannot meet the measures without viable portal solutions, so they are pressuring the EMR and portal vendors for more workable options.

Without a perfect solution at present, health care organizations are advised to work closely with their legal counsel and health information management staff to ensure the access given through a portal complies with their state's own unique regulations. Providers must communicate the details of access policies regarding patient portals for younger patients. All stipulations should be clearly stated in an authorization or terms-of-use form that parents agree to prior to gaining access to their child's information in the portal.[12]

THE CHALLENGE OF CONFIDENTIALITY WITH PATIENT PORTALS

Of the many challenges that exist when implementing a patient portal for the child and adolescent population, none is so prevalent or widely discussed as those related to confidentiality. Confidentiality remains a major reason that many teenagers forgo much-needed care in their own lives.[14] It stands to reason that while patient portals present a mechanism by which adolescent patients can interface with their physicians, they also present a potential pitfall for breaches of confidentiality between teens and their parents.

Attitudes and opinions regarding confidentiality in patient portals are well documented in the literature.[9,15–18] Survey studies examining confidentiality in adolescent portals show low parental concern for maintaining the confidentiality of their children's information as it relates to parental access.[18] Interestingly, 1e area in which parents have expressed some concern is the possibility of their own comments regarding their children spoken to providers being shared with teens through access granted in patient portals.[9] Expectedly, teenagers feel strongly that patient portals need to maintain confidentiality in regards to their health and wish to remain autonomous in some important areas of medical decision making.[11] Discrepancies do exist between younger and older adolescent opinions about confidentiality. In general, younger patients worry about other health care providers seeing sensitive information and express a desire for parental involvement in their care. Older adolescents tend to worry about information being shared with their parents and want that information kept confidential.[17]

Given the shift in attitudes regarding confidentiality through child/adolescent development and the sensitive nature of health care issues prevalent among older adolescents, patient portals should be flexible in their ability to grant or restrict access based on preference and age of any given patient. Although patients may welcome and need parental involvement and access to patient portals in childhood and early adolescence, portals generally should have access policies that change for patients as they age through adolescence and into adulthood.

UTILIZATION AND PARENT/TEEN OPINION OF PATIENT PORTALS

When patient portals are built and instituted, there is no guarantee that they will be used. In fact, data regarding the utilization of child and adolescent patient portals show that there are some interesting patterns regarding utilization. Some studies have shown a fairly significant discrepancy in activation and enrollment of patient portal accounts within the EMR. Certain factors, including ethnicity and socioeconomic status, seemed to be predictive variables of utilization, with a lower utilization in Medicaid populations, lower socioeconomic status, and certain minority groups.[19] Although the data show some interesting discrepancies in utilization data between different ethnic and cultural groups, there are few data investigating the opinions or attitudes regarding EMRs, portals, and confidentiality that might help explain these discrepancies. Further research into this area is needed.

Utilization was higher for patients with chronic diagnoses including autism.[20] This points out the importance of availability of these portals for patients with chronic mental health conditions.

Published literature reviewing utilization data shows that enrollment for adolescent patient portal accounts ranges anywhere from 4% to 65% of patients. Activation (logging in at least once) of these accounts ranges anywhere from 26% to 29%.[2] One study showed an enrollment of 28%, with 48% of those patients logging onto the portal at least 1 time, and 16% of those patients continuing to use the portal in the coming weeks and months.[20] Utilization data show that, in general, parents tend to use portals more than their teenagers.[2]

As one might expect, there is a fairly significant disparity between parent opinion and adolescent opinion when it comes to the utilization of patient portals for child and adolescent patients.[19]

For the most part, parents liked the idea of portals for their children.[10] They liked the facilitated communication that the portals offer with providers, but did not see it as a replacement for direct communication with the providers.[18,21] They found that access to their children's information provided reduced anxiety and reassurance, but also expressed concern about learning details of new diagnoses or other anxiety-provoking information, for which they preferred direct communication.[22] Parents in many of the studies reviewed for this article felt that institutions should require parental consent before their teenagers are able to access patient portals. A recurring theme throughout the literature is that parents do not want to be left out of the loop when it comes to the care of their children.[11]

Unsurprisingly, teenagers also have fairly strong opinions regarding patient portals. Generally, teenagers want to be in control of their own health care.[11] In the studies reviewed, teens were enthusiastic to have access to their providers and scheduling, which provoked some anxiety in parents. Teens expressed anxiety about their parents having access to patient portals, and the subject most pervasively present throughout the literature was that of the importance of confidentiality.

DISCUSSION

With all of the complexities surrounding portal access for adolescence, it is not unreasonable to wonder if it is really worth the effort. Do teenagers really want electronic access to their health care information? A recent study by Pew Research Center, titled "Teens, Social Media & Technology Overview 2015" found that 92% of teens aged 13 to 17 report going online daily and that nearly three-quarters of them have or have access to a smart phone (**Fig. 1**).[23] Online access has become an ingrained part of social behavior for teens, so it makes sense to interface with teens in the most natural way possible: electronically!

Another 2015 study, led by Ellen Wartella of Northwestern University, found that 84% of teens aged 13 to 18 surf the Internet when they want answers to questions about their health. Ellen stated, "Half the teens who use search engines to look for health information say they usually just click on the first site that comes up."[24] This is an area where a portal catering to adolescents could have the potential to offer evidence-based education regarding health. Allowing teens with mental health concerns easy access to reliable information, avoiding the stigma and misinformation

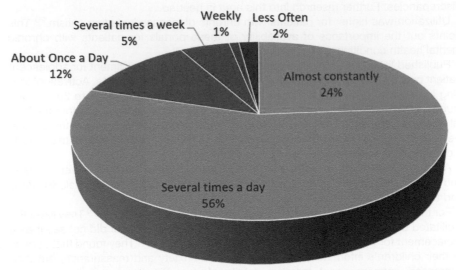

% of teens ages 13–17 who use the internet with the following frequencies

Several times a week
5%

Weekly
1%

Less Often
2%

About Once a Day
12%

Almost constantly
24%

Several times a day
56%

Fig. 1. Frequency of Internet use by teens. (*Data from* Lenhart A. Teens, social media & technology overview 2015. Pew Res Cent Internet Sci Tech; 2015. Available at: http://www.pewinternet.org/2015/04/09/teens-social-media-technology-2015/. Accessed May 25, 2016.)

pervasive in society and the Internet, has exciting potential implications. How many more teens might ask their regular physician a health question if it was as easy to do as posting a status update on their favorite social media application?

Although much of this article has focused on the use of patient portals for child and adolescent patients in general, there are aspects of their use in child and adolescent psychiatry that bear more in-depth evaluation. The ability for parents and teenagers to communicate directly with their children's mental health provider opens up valuable, but also potentially complicated scenarios. For instance, patients of mental health providers often experience acute periods of crisis that require emergent intervention. Use of the patient portal for these instances could potentially lead to unnecessary and potential dangerous delay in care. Survey data of parents and teenagers show that both agree that the portal should not be used for emergent mental health issues.[11]

The discussions in this article regarding confidentiality obviously extend to the treatment of psychiatric patients. The introduction of the EMR and its use in psychiatric practice has justifiably raised some concern about its impact on the doctor–patient relationship. Confidentiality between providers and their child adolescent patients is often paramount to this relationship. Given the complex nature of mental health record systems and their accompanying patient portals, there is no perfect mechanism to correctly identify sensitive information to be withheld 100% of the time. There are bound to be mistakes. Providers should have open communication with their young patients and the guardians of these patients about the use of patient portals in their practice and the potential risks inherent to their use. Practices should develop policies on how to address potential breaches of confidentiality should they arise and understand the potential effect this may have on the rapport and trust in their therapeutic relationships.

Discussions surrounding confidentiality, especially between teenagers and parents, may introduce opportunities to facilitate and develop communication skills and strategies and thus therapeutic benefit to the parent–child relationship. As described earlier in the article, there are often significant discrepancies in opinion as to what information should be withheld or not withheld regarding adolescent mental health. Helping patients and parents come to an agreement or understanding of institutional policy only serves to strengthen communication skills during a potentially rocky time for teens and their parents.

SUMMARY

It is only fitting that in an era emphasizing and facilitating increased autonomy for patients regarding their own health care, technologies such as patient portals should be accessed by young patients who themselves are navigating a period of development for which autonomy is a major milestone. Helping child and adolescent patients understand and utilize the tools that patient portals can provide facilitates and engenders participation and engagement in the management of their own mental health. Although confidentiality issues inherent to the practice of psychiatry with younger patients are further complicated by the institution of patient portals, the careful institution of well thought out policies and open communication with patients helps mitigate potential risk. The use of patient portals in child and adolescent psychiatry offers numerous benefits to both providers and patients, and represents an exciting and engaging way in which physicians interface with those for whom they care.

REFERENCES

1. What is a patient portal? Available at: https://www.healthit.gov/providers-professionals/faqs/what-patient-portal. Accessed May 22, 2016.
2. Bush RA, Connelly CD, Fuller M, et al. Implementation of the integrated electronic patient portal in the pediatric population: a systematic review. Telemed J E Health 2015. http://dx.doi.org/10.1089/tmj.2015.0033.
3. 7 Portals Powering Patient Engagement. InformationWeek. Available at: http://www.informationweek.com/healthcare/clinical-systems/7-portals-powering-patient-engagement/240147137. Accessed May 25, 2016.
4. Medicare C for, Baltimore MS 7500 SB, USA M. 2016Programrequirements. 2016. Available at: https://www.cms.gov/Regulations-and-Guidance/Legislation/EHRIncentivePrograms/2016ProgramRequirements.html. Accessed May 25, 2016.
5. OpenNotes. Available at: http://www.opennotes.org/. Accessed May 22, 2016.
6. Who is sharing notes? OpenNotes. Available at: http://www.opennotes.org/who-is-sharing-notes/. Accessed May 22, 2016.
7. Vodicka E, Mejilla R, Leveille SG, et al. Online access to doctors' notes: patient concerns about privacy. J Med Internet Res 2013;15(9):e208.
8. Dobscha SK, Denneson LM, Jacobson LE, et al. VA mental health clinician experiences and attitudes toward opennotes. Gen Hosp Psychiatry 2016;38:89–93.
9. Bourgeois FC, Taylor PL, Emans SJ, et al. Whose personal control? Creating private, personally controlled health records for pediatric and adolescent patients. J Am Med Inform Assoc 2008;15(6):737–43.
10. Ahlers-Schmidt CR, Nguyen M. Parent intention to use a patient portal as related to their children following a facilitated demonstration. Telemed J E Health 2013;19(12):979–81.

11. Bergman DA, Brown NL, Wilson S. Teen use of a patient portal: a qualitative study of parent and teen attitudes. Perspect Health Inf Manag 2008;5:13.
12. Office for Civil Rights. Does the HIPAA privacy rule allow parents the right to see their children's medical records? HHS.gov. 2015. Available at: http://www.hhs.gov/hipaa/for-professionals/faq/227/can-i-access-medical-record-if-i-have-power-of-attorney/index.html. Accessed May 25, 2016.
13. Dimitropoulos L. Privacy and Security Solutions for Interoperable Health Information Exchange. 2009. Available at: https://www.healthit.gov/sites/default/files/patient-matching-white-paper-final-2.pdf. Accessed May 25, 2016.
14. Eytan T, Hereford J. Patients, physicians, and the internet. Manag Care Q 2002; 10(1):11–5.
15. Ford C, English A, Sigman G. Confidential health care for adolescents: position paper for the society for adolescent medicine. J Adolesc Health 2004;35(2): 160–7.
16. Informed consent, parental permission, and assent in pediatric practice. Committee on Bioethics, American Academy of Pediatrics. Pediatrics 1995;95(2):314–7.
17. Britto MT, Tivorsak TL, Slap GB. Adolescents' needs for health care privacy. Pediatrics 2010;126(6):e1469–1476.
18. Byczkowski TL, Munafo JK, Britto MT. Family perceptions of the usability and value of chronic disease web-based patient portals. Health Inform J 2014; 20(2):151–62.
19. Ketterer T, West DW, Sanders VP, et al. Correlates of patient portal enrollment and activation in primary care pediatrics. Acad Pediatr 2013;13(3):264–71.
20. Byczkowski TL, Munafo JK, Britto MT. Variation in use of Internet-based patient portals by parents of children with chronic disease. Arch Pediatr Adolesc Med 2011;165(5):405–11.
21. Britto MT, Jimison HB, Munafo JK, et al. Usability testing finds problems for novice users of pediatric portals. J Am Med Inform Assoc 2009;16(5):660–9.
22. Britto MT, Hesse EA, Kamdar OJ, et al. Parents' perceptions of a patient portal for managing their child's chronic illness. J Pediatr 2013;163(1):280–1.e1-2.
23. Lenhart A. Teens, social media & technology overview 2015. Washington, DC: Pew Res Cent Internet Sci Tech; 2015. Available at: http://www.pewinternet.org/2015/04/09/teens-social-media-technology-2015/. Accessed May 25, 2016.
24. Kelly M. Majority of teens surf the web for answers to health questions. Live Science. Available at: http://www.livescience.com/51042-teens-health-information-internet.html. Accessed May 25, 2016.

Transformational Impact of Health Information Technology on the Clinical Practice of Child and Adolescent Psychiatry

Todd E. Peters, MD

KEYWORDS

- Health information technology • Child and adolescent psychiatry
- Medical informatics • Health IT • Pediatric behavioral health care
- Clinical decision support

KEY POINTS

- Child and adolescent psychiatrists are faced with many challenges in implementing health information technology strategies, such as electronic health records, into clinical practice. These challenges have likely contributed to a delay in implementation within psychiatry.
- Several strategies can be implemented to improve patient care using health information technology, including clinical decision support strategies integrated with electronic health record systems.
- Future growth within behavioral health information technology will be imperative to align with other medical specialties in the multidisciplinary care of youth. Reaching a balance between privacy and increased transparency of care will be imperative.

INTRODUCTION

This is an exciting but difficult time for treating mental health needs in youth. In treating the pediatric population, no child or adolescent now knows of a time without cellular phones or widespread Internet use. According to Pew Research Center data from 2015, 92% of teenagers access the Internet daily and 73% have regular access to smartphone devices. Most teenagers also regularly access social media sites, which have become a major source of news and information for teens. In some ways, this movement has likely assisted with destigmatization of mental health issues in in the

Disclosure: The author has nothing to disclose.
Department of Psychiatry and Behavioral Sciences, Vanderbilt Psychiatric Hospital, Vanderbilt University Medical Center, 1601 23rd Avenue South, Nashville, TN 37212-8645, USA
E-mail address: Todd.peters@vanderbilt.edu

Child Adolesc Psychiatric Clin N Am 26 (2017) 55–66
http://dx.doi.org/10.1016/j.chc.2016.07.003
1056-4993/17/© 2016 Elsevier Inc. All rights reserved.

United States, giving millions of youth and their families a platform to share struggles with psychiatric symptoms and treatment. However, children's use of social media can give them access to millions of people at their fingertips, which offers significant risk, including the inherent risk of more widespread bullying, sexual exploitation, and discussion of self-injury or suicide strategies.

Although children have been quick to adopt the latest technological advances in treatment, many child and adolescent behavioral health practitioners have been slow to adopt health information technology (IT) in their clinical practice. Studies have shown that psychiatrists are the least likely to adopt use of electronic health records (EHRs) in clinical practice. Although previously many providers questioned whether to have a Web site for their practice or accept emails from patients, now providers are faced with pressures to respond to negative Yelp or Google ratings by frustrated patients or to have their own social media presence. Given these advances in health information and the expansive use of the Internet by most patients and families, practitioners are faced with a challenge unlike those faced in preceding generations. How do practitioners discuss the use of electronic communication between providers/institutions and electronic medical records with patients, recognizing that the patients/families are the true owners of their medical records?

Although it is sometimes easier to focus on the potential pitfalls of practicing in the Internet/digital age, this article takes a more balanced approach in focusing on the transformational nature of health IT, including:

1. Optimizing use of EHRs for clinical practice, including documentation strategies to improve care
2. Leveraging health IT to improve quality of care, especially through clinical decision support (CDS) strategies and electronic standardized assessments
3. Focusing on potential for future growth in the realm of health IT in child and adolescent psychiatric practice

BACKGROUND FOR HEALTH INFORMATION TECHNOLOGY IN CHILD PSYCHIATRIC PRACTICE

The area of clinical documentation is not a new challenge in psychiatry. Historically, issues surrounding information that should be documented in the legal medical record, including the personal and private details of each patient's personal history, have challenged providers. Documentation of practitioners' work continues to serve many purposes: to serve as an internal record of patient care; to detail evaluations and assessments for other providers within a health care team; to justify the work that is performed for billing/insurance; and to serve as an external record for families, especially in times of litigation. Historically, many providers have incorrectly thought that a patient's medical chart is the property of the practice or provider, creating barriers to open access by the patients. Over time, most practitioners have come to understand that, although providers are the legal creators of the record, the patient remains the true owner. In child and adolescent practice, this delineation is unclear and depends on the state laws where each clinician practices.

Safety and confidentiality issues are also not new to the digital age. However, this has become exacerbated with the advent of remotely accessible EHR systems, especially in mental health. Because of these concerns for confidentiality, the Health Insurance Portability and Accountability Act (HIPAA) was created in 1996 to provide additional regulations for so-called covered entities, which are any practices or institutions that perform electronic transfer of clinical information. After this development, signed disclosure statements releasing electronic dissemination of documents became essential.[1] The advent of the digital age has led to more widespread use of EHRs, assisted by the Health Information Technology for Economic and Clinical Health (HITECH) Act, which incentivized the use of EHR-based systems in clinical practice. The increasing use of EHRs has prioritized the development of linkages between EHRs systems in the form of health information exchanges (HIEs). These exchanges offer significant improvement in aspects of patient care and safety but also open a wider window for security breaches and access to potentially sensitive information by external providers and staff. However, the complexities of integration between hundreds of available EHR vendors have slowed the process of data sharing within HIEs. Recent studies continue to show that significant barriers exist to prevent optimal sharing of patient information between providers and institution.[2]

Although behavioral health providers have struggled with health IT adoption, there have been other factors that have impaired growth. Many behavioral health providers were excluded from initial government incentives for EHR adoption because of stringent criteria for physicians.[3] In addition, many larger institutions and academic centers have been challenged with integration of mental health records into system-wide EHR platforms in an effort to ensure continued privacy of the sensitive information that is often detailed within mental health records. In addition, for those who treat patients struggling with substance abuse issues, many laws prevent or curtail incorporation of these issues into central problem lists on patient medical records. These concerns and previous legal precedents have slowed the full integration of mental health issues into medical homes or multidisciplinary treatment environments.

Difficulties with mental health information integration can be further exacerbated when working with youth. In most medical settings, parents have direct access to their children's medical records until they turn 18 years of age or are legally emancipated. However, this is more complicated with behavioral health treatment records. There is potential risk to allowing full access of minors' mental health information to their parents or legal guardians. When addressing these issues, it is imperative to review the relevant state laws to determine what information is protected within behavioral health records.[4,5] In addition, it is essential to understand the process of blocking or sequestering extremely sensitive information within the legal medical record within the EHR, such as therapy process notes or information that could lead to potential emotional or physical trauma for the patients. Given these challenges, it is understandable that psychiatrists, especially child and adolescent mental health providers, have been slow to adopt EHRs[6-8] and are the specialists with some of the lowest rates of overall EHR use.[9] Other barriers to EHR use, such as disruption to workflow, more limited eye contact, missed visual cues from patients, and decreased time with patients,[10-15] have also stymied growth of behavioral health IT use.

However, to avoid adoption of EHR use and other health IT advances stands to keep behavioral health providers on the periphery of the advances in medicine. In addition, child and adolescent psychiatrists' work within accountable care organizations and medical home models may be limited without more global adoptions of EHRs. Mental health practitioners' concerns about a drastically altered form of clinical practice are often not realized, as shown by research dating back to the 1990s. One of the first articles studied the beliefs of providers after EHR implementation, which showed that most providers thought that the content and quality of patient interactions were preserved with EHR use.[16] Another postimplementation study at Vanderbilt University studied mental health providers' views of the impact of EHR use 1 year after initiation. This study found that therapeutic communication with patients was maintained and that notes were clearer and more legible. However, most of these providers struggled with documentation around confidential information within the electronic medical record, even when these records were sequestered in their own psychiatric database.[17]

OPTIMIZING DOCUMENTATION IN THE DIGITAL AGE

The need to balance confidentiality and transparency in the medical record is not a new issue with EHR use. However, EHRs provide the ability to more easily access the medical records of patients by others within a health system, between health systems through HIEs, or by patients/family members through electronic health portals. Many child and adolescent mental health providers have struggled with maintaining the safety of the patients and families that they treat.[18] Historical information, such as mental health issues within family histories, details around divorce within social histories, and descriptions of family dynamics within patient notes, can have significant impact on the care of the children being treated, such as in custody disputes and contentious separations between carers. Given these downstream implications, coupled with greater ease of access, many providers have adjusted their documentation styles within EHRs.[19]

All documentation should occur with the understanding that the child or guardian will eventually read the note and visualize the full record for the treatment course.[20–22] Given this guiding principal, one main strategy is to document the smallest amount of information possible to allow care coordination and billing.[23] This strategy includes clinicians practicing only within their scope of practice and avoiding disclosure of other providers' documentation/notes.[20] In addition, it is imperative to allow for time within patient appointments to discuss diagnoses and details that will be charted within the legal medical record. This time minimizes concern by patients when they access their records after care has been provided.

Many EHR care portals allow for access to laboratory work, communication tools, scheduled appointments, and some patient care notes/details. However, most currently struggle with how to address access to mental health treatment information within these portals. At this time, most behavioral health notes are excluded from patient portals or are sequestered in separate mental health databases within EHR systems. In the near future, many EHR vendors are moving toward full transparency of patient records. Meaningful-use requirements are pushing for more transparency of patient records through electronic portals. Driving this movement are research findings from many providers and institutions who have given patients full access to their medical records, including notes detailing mental health care. In one of the largest studies to date, entitled OpenNotes, more than 20,000 patients were given access to their entire medical records through an electronic health portal in 3 separate care settings.[24,25] This 1-year study encompassed the clinical practices of more than 100 primary care providers. After the study period, patients could continue open access if they chose to do so. During the study period, more than 13,000 patients accessed at least 1 note within their medical records.[24] Most patients thought that they had more control of their care and were subjectively more compliant with their medication regimens. However, approximately 30% of patients voiced that this improved access heightened their worries about privacy issues. Despite many providers' fears before enrollment, there was no discernable change to the number of electronic messages sent by patients who were enrolled in the study to their providers. In addition, most providers did not think that this change greatly altered their documentation practices aside from potential increase in documentation time (up to 21%) and slight alteration to the content of information documented. Despite these slight impacts in workflow, no providers wished to withdraw their access after the 1-year study period and 99% of patients continued full access.[25,26]

This ground-breaking research has led some mental health providers to push for greater transparency and open access of mental health records as well.[26] These providers hypothesize that institutions and individual providers have concern that information detailed in mental health treatment notes may be traumatic for patients and may curtail open discussion of mental health issues moving forward. Instead, these providers argue that open access will instead allow for more open communication around mental health issues, giving their patients the opportunity to review their records in their home environments in a less pressured situation. However, they also recognize that full access to all information has limitations as well. They support the idea that some clinical information should be able to be marked as excluded from these portals if deemed potentially harmful or destabilizing for their patients. These researchers summarized their recommendations with the following statement: "By writing notes useful to both patients and ourselves and then inviting them to read what we write, we may help patients address their mental health issues more actively and reduce the stigma they experience."[26]

As practitioners become more transparent with clinical documentation, it is imperative to use techniques to make documentation more understandable to the patients who read them. Historically, patient notes have served as a communication tool between providers. These notes are often laden with complex medical terminologies and diagnoses that are often recognizable only by those in the field. However, this format is counter to the patient care movement, which is centered on the understanding that the owner of the medical record, the patient, is often not trained in medicine. In turn, some providers have pushed for removal of complex medical jargon, to be replaced by more common, everyday language.[27] Some have lobbied for summarizing care and diagnostic formulations into a more condensed form. This so-called medical tweet would allow a more descriptive, nonjudgmental summary of patient care that could demystify the work that clinicians do as a profession and could work to destigmatize psychiatry as a whole.[27] The focus on a more succinct formulation could also curtail so-called note bloat, in which information is copied and pasted from note to note, which unnecessarily lengthens notes and creates potential confusion about the care that was provided, especially if contradictory information is present in the same note.

Medical documentation within health records often prioritizes positive symptoms pointing to disease or underlying diagnoses. This focus often causes patient strengths and resiliency factors to be overlooked. Detailing these strengths is especially important when working with youth.[26] Many children and adolescents the authors treat think that they are stuck in home environments that focus more on their disorders than their positive factors and traits. Giving equal focus to strengths and resiliency factors can assist with initiation of therapy and delineate a clearer path toward health. This strategy also helps to make patients feel more like people instead of patients.

Another strategy to improve clarity of documentation is to avoid hedge phrases in clinical documentation.[28] This issue is not new to EHR use, but has the potential to become more of an issue with greater access by patients to their treatment notes. Mental health providers have shown high levels of these phrases in clinical documentation, which may stem from fear of making declarative diagnostic impressions caused by stigma associated with certain diagnoses or fear of legal ramifications from incorrect diagnoses. However, these phrases often lead to greater ambiguity and misinterpretations by patients, which can lead to poorer outcomes related to patient-provider relationships/trust. These hedge phrases may show the struggle that psychiatry has in applying rigid Diagnostic and Statistical Manual of Mental Disorders (DSM) diagnoses to patients, especially constantly developing youth. However, being more transparent in documentation of diagnostic uncertainty may lead to overall improvements in future communication and may enhance the overall satisfaction with the patient-provider relationship.[29–32]

Several studies have shown potential clinical care benefits with increased transparency. Patients with substance use issues often delay care for more than 10 years after initial substance use,[33] which often first occurs in adolescence. Use of an EHR system may allow better tracking of substance use across the multidisciplinary care team.[34] Extrapolating these data, tracking other mental health disorders may be successful as well. Other internalizing disorders, such as anxiety/obsessive-compulsive disorder, eating disorders, and depression, have a similar pattern of delay with reporting and could be better reported through shared EHR systems.

ELECTRONIC CLINICAL DECISION SUPPORT FOR MENTAL HEALTH TREATMENT

One of the main factors that prompt providers to transition to EHR use is the allure of using electronic CDS systems in their clinical practices.

When most providers think of CDS, they envision typing information into the EHR system as part of their documentation workflow, which will trigger treatment strategies and alerts based on evidence-based treatment algorithms embedded in the electronic system. As described by the Centers for Medicare and Medicaid Services (CMS), CDS is composed of various tools to improve quality of care and health outcomes. These tools include computerized alerts and reminders for both providers and patients, clinical guidelines for care, condition-specific order sets, templates for documentation, patient data reports, and diagnostic support. As detailed within the CMS Five Rights concept, CDS interventions allow the right information to be available to the right people through the right channels in the right intervention formats at the right points in the workflow.[35] CDS systems serve as customizable toolboxes that can be optimized by the clinical practice, institution, or end user, depending on the setup of the system and practice. Some CDS tools include clinical knowledge bases, which are treatment algorithms derived from best-practice strategies, drug formularies, and drug interaction tools. CDS systems were a main driver for the HITECH incentive programs designed to transition practices to digital documentation, with the hope that the quality of medical care would be improved.[36] Over the last 2 decades, many studies and review articles have attempted to test the long-held belief that use of EHR and CDS systems would enhance quality of care. However, the results of these review studies have been mixed,[37] with many studies showing improvement in outcomes with regard to diagnosis, disease management, prescribing behaviors, and practitioner performance,[38,39] whereas other studies have shown no consistent association between CDS use and quality outcomes.[36]

These varied results may be caused by CDS strategies serving more as a toolbox than as a physician's clinical assistant. Just as a carpenter should not blame the hammer for missing a nail, practitioners should not blame a CDS system for missing quality metrics, especially if the correct settings and algorithms are not in place to do so. In order to maximize the quality of results, continued practice with each tool is essential to leverage quality outcomes. Most EHR/CDS systems are designed with too many alerts, which can lead to end-user alert fatigue and changes in workflow.[40] This fatigue can lead providers to ignore or overlook more essential alerts/indications amid the noise of other alerts. In turn, it is important to hone the CDS system as much as possible to preserve essential alerts. When selecting a CDS vendor or developing CDS tools, it is imperative to have the ability to execute more granular control of messages and alerts received, applicable to the clinical setting of each practice.

CDS systems have been studied in clinical practice within psychiatry. However, as in many other areas of health IT, psychiatry has lagged behind other medical and surgical fields. A likely contributor to this lack of research in psychiatry is the complexity of mental health diagnoses, which often rely on complex, multitiered, subjective data rather than numbers-based objective data, which are primarily used in other medical fields. Given this complexity, most of the research has centered on studies aiding in standardized diagnostic assessments. These assessments, such as the Structured Clinical Interview for DSM (SCID), have been used in clinical practice and research for many decades. However, the transition to electronic formats of these well-studied tools has been problematic at times. The Computer-Based Structured Clinical Interview for DSM-IV (CB-SCID1), a CDS that is an electronic form of the SCID, was developed to facilitate the proper DSM diagnosis or diagnoses after automatically tabulating met criteria. However, embedded strategies to facilitate and automate the process led to automation bias, which then caused issues with errors of omission and commission that at times compromised the diagnostic results.[41] Several studies have shown significant disagreement between diagnoses rendered from clinician-based evaluations versus more computerized/automated systems.[41] In some studies comparing International Classification of Diseases, 10th Revision (ICD-10) agreement, results were as low as 56%.[42]

Many studies have examined the use of CDS strategies for diagnostic assessment in clinical settings (outpatient and emergency departments).[43–46] These studies measured quality through several practitioner performance outcomes, such as rate of referrals to outpatient mental health providers, appropriate screening of mood disorders (especially depressive disorders), and proper use of antidepressants for depressed patients. However, these early studies did not show a robust effect on practitioner performance and patient outcomes, as measured by symptom severity score after several weeks to months.[38,43–46]

Other studies on CDS tools in psychiatry have focused on a more systematic approach to monitoring depression diagnosis and severity in clinical settings.[47] Many of these systems use the freely available Nine-Item Patient Health Questionnaire (PHQ-9) for regular assessment of clinical severity of depressive symptoms with each clinical visit.[48] Other systems have taken these regular assessments a step further by electronically mapping treatment algorithm for depression.[49] One such program electronically mapped the Texas Medication Algorithm Project (TMAP)[50] into a more automated, computerized format (CompTMAP).[51] Previous studies had shown that patients treated for major depressive disorder in the TMAP showed better outcomes than those who received treatment as usual within the clinical settings studied. The CompTMAP program focused on electronic decision support to ascertain the appropriate diagnosis and then recommended treatment choices, follow-up frequency, and preventive care strategies.[51] Electronic diagnostic and treatment tools such as CompTMAP are being developed and used in psychiatric clinical practice, but outcomes data have been sparse to date.

As described previously, psychiatry, especially child and adolescent psychiatry, is lagging behind in CDS systems research. However, it is essential that child and adolescent psychiatrists progress as rapidly as possible to improve quality of care to better manage longitudinal risk for pediatric patients with mental health issues. An often missed opportunity to improve risk outcomes is to assess and document a structured risk assessment of patients seeking psychiatric treatment. Based on research published by the US Centers for Disease Control and Prevention, there were 42,773 deaths by suicide in the United States in 2014. Suicide is the 10th leading cause of death in all ages. It remains the second leading cause of death for people 15 to 24 years old.[52] However,

Milton and colleagues[53] showed that suicide risk assessments were completed in only 38% of individuals who later committed suicide. Developing strategies to use EHR/CDS systems to help systematize safety assessments is imperative. Triggering alerts for completion of risk assessments for patients at risk would be an invaluable tool for use in clinical practice. Taking this one step further, many EHR systems allow for electronic screening and questionnaire completion in the waiting room or via secure e-mail before the patient's appointment. These screening measures can be vital in child and adolescent psychiatry, because many patients are uncomfortable discussing safety issues in the presence of their carers. These discrete data points can then be securely uploaded into the EHR for clinical assessment, decision support, and data tracking. However, given the large amount of data available in most EHR systems, important information such as safety assessment metrics can become lost. Biomedical informatics will continue to be essential in this area. Comparative effectiveness research can use visual analytics to ensure that vital information needed for CDS is readily available and more rapidly interpreted to aid in treatment approaches and outcomes measurement.[54,55] Future development in this and other areas of psychiatric practice will undoubtedly save lives and improve patient outcomes.

SUMMARY/DISCUSSION OF FUTURE PSYCHIATRIC HEALTH INFORMATION TECHNOLOGY RESEARCH STRATEGIES AND GOALS

The digital age is here. Most child and adolescent psychiatric providers accept this fact, readily adopting the latest smartphone, tablet, operating system, or social media platform. However, many child and adolescent psychiatrists think that they are being forced to use EHRs and other electronic treatment strategies in clinical practice by government mandates or by their employers. The time has come (and has nearly passed) for medical providers to fully adopt EHRs in their clinical practice. Also, implementing separate EHR systems from other medical providers within an organization can also lead to difficulties with interoperability and double documentation.[56] Further delay in implementation places child and adolescent psychiatry at risk of being left behind in the evolving world of medical homes and accountable care organizations, many of which are structured and united by a shared electronic medical record to improve collaborative decision-making approaches to patient care. It is imperative that all providers educate themselves on EHR systems and associated policies that directly affect implementation and use.

The landscape of psychiatric practice has also evolved over the years, as clearly shown by the progression and evolution of the DSM since its inception. Changing the way child and adolescent psychiatrists document and communicate psychiatric diagnoses/treatment is just as important as changing the understanding of diagnostic criteria associated with these diagnoses. Given that child and adolescent psychiatrists are often seen as experts in development, these same providers need to develop as well, adjusting practice styles and techniques to better meet the needs of their patients.

Medicine is moving toward a more patient-centered care model built on transparency and more open access to the health record. Historically, the mental health field has been wary to accept transparency, let alone full disclosure of mental health treatment notes. Based on multiple treatment studies, patients will welcome transparency of mental health care. Actively discussing information listed in progress notes and the rationale for treatment will create dialogue that will help to destigmatize mental health diagnoses and treatment. Continuing to routinely sequester mental health information within medical records will hinder psychiatry moving forward. For child and adolescent providers, advocating for patients and families and working collaboratively with other medical providers to improve the overall health of patients will be vital. By improving research strategies and IT implementation, psychiatrists can close the gap between theirs and other medical professions.

Future areas of research and growth should be multifaceted. From a public policy and privacy standpoint, child and adolescent psychiatrists would benefit from further strategies to improve flow of necessary mental health data (eg, medications, treatment) between EHR systems while actively participating in the creation of policies protecting sensitive information about youth. Psychiatrists should also advocate for standards associated with patient portals for minors, delineating who has access to sensitive information available within these access points. As the medical field moves toward more transparency of patient care notes, future research will be essential to monitor the effects of additional transparency between minor patients and their carers. Adopting an approach in behavioral health similar to the OpenNotes study may help to keep psychiatry relevant in the evolving landscape of medical care.

From a behavioral health IT perspective, further research on electronic, standardized approaches to diagnosis and care through CDS systems will benefit child and adolescent psychiatry. Continued education in health technology should remain a central focus of specialty conferences and other continued medical education opportunities. The use of electronic tools to track safety metrics and suicide risk factors in youth has the potential to improve clinical outcomes and reduce mortality. In addition, social media platforms have become the "experts" for many youth in coping with and managing suicidal thoughts and safety issues. Learning more from this phenomenon will help child and adolescent psychiatry advance as well.

Overall, this is a difficult but exciting time to be a child and adolescent psychiatrist. Embracing the transformative impact of health IT instead of running or hiding from its shortcomings will help child and adolescent psychiatry remain viable in a changing treatment landscape. During this time of transition, providers must align with government standards and public policy to stay relevant. Psychiatry will also benefit from further alignment with other medical specialties to best care for the population as a whole. Only then can psychiatry reach parity with other medical specialties.

REFERENCES

1. Houston M. The psychiatric medical record, HIPAA, and the use of electronic medical records. Child Adolesc Psychiatr Clin N Am 2010;19(1):107–14.
2. Quigley L, Lacombe-Duncan A, Adams S, et al. A qualitative analysis of information sharing for children with medical complexity within and across health care organizations. BMC Health Serv Res 2014;14:283.
3. Miller JE, Glover RW, Gordon SY. Crossing the behavioral health digital divide: the role of health information technology in improving care for people with serious mental illness in state mental health systems. 2014. Available at: http://www.nasmhpd.org/content/crossing-behavioral-health-digital-divide-role-health-information-technology-improving-care. Accessed June 26, 2016.
4. Mandl KD, Szolovits P, Kohane IS. Public standards and patients' control: how to keep electronic medical records accessible but private. BMJ 2001;322(7281):283–7.
5. HIPAA facts: parent and minor rights. Provided by the Technical Assistance Support Center of the National Association for Rights Protection & Advocacy. Q&A by Susan Stefan, Center for Public Representation. Available at: http://unitedcivilrights.org/members/HIPAA/HIPAA-parent-info1.pdf. Accessed June 26, 2016.

6. Lefkovitz PM. Behavioral health/human services information systems survey: executive summary/media release. 2009. Available at: http://www.satva.org/documents/InformationSystemsSurveyReportFinal.pdf. Accessed June 26, 2016.

7. Mojtabai R. Datapoints: use of information technology by psychiatrists and other medical providers. Psychiatr Serv 2007;58(10):1261.

8. Hsiao C, Beatty PC, Hing ES, et al. Electronic medical record/electronic health record use by office-based physicians: United States, 2008 and preliminary 2009. Available at: http://www.cdc.gov/nchs/data/hestat/emr_ehr/emr_ehr.pdf. Accessed June 26, 2016.

9. Burt CW, Sisk JE. Which physicians and practices are using electronic medical records? Health Aff (Millwood) 2005;24(5):1334–43.

10. Stewart RF, Kroth PJ, Schuyler M, et al. Do electronic health records affect the patient-psychiatrist relationship? A before & after study of psychiatric outpatients. BMC Psychiatry 2010;10:3.

11. Makoul G, Curry RH, Tang PC. The use of electronic medical records: communication patterns in outpatient encounters. J Am Med Inform Assoc 2001;8(6):610–5.

12. Linder JA, Schnipper JL, Tsurikova R, et al. Barriers to electronic health record use during patient visits. AMIA Annu Symp Proc 2006;499–503.

13. Chaudhry B, Wang J, Wu S, et al. Systematic review: impact of health information technology on quality, efficiency, and costs of medical care. Ann Intern Med 2006;144(10):742–52.

14. Baron RJ, Fabens EL, Schiffman M, et al. Electronic health records: just around the corner? or over the cliff? Ann Intern Med 2005;143(3):222–6.

15. Jaspers MW, Knaup P, Schmidt D. The computerized patient record: where do we stand? Yearb Med Inform 2006;29–39. Available at: http://imia.schattauer.de/en/contents/archive/issue/2254.html. Accessed September 18, 2016.

16. Marshall PD, Chin HL. The effects of an electronic medical record on patient care: clinician attitudes in a large HMO. Proc AMIA Symp 1998;150–4.

17. Salomon RM, Blackford JU, Rosenbloom ST, et al. Openness of patients' reporting with use of electronic records: psychiatric clinicians' views. J Am Med Inform Assoc 2010;17(1):54–60.

18. Chiu SH, Fitzgerald KM. Electronic medical/health record and pediatric behavioral health providers: progress and problems. Arch Psychiatr Nurs 2013;27(2):108–9.

19. Nielsen BA, Baum RA, Soares NS. Navigating ethical issues with electronic health records in developmental-behavioral pediatric practice. J Dev Behav Pediatr 2013;34(1):45–51.

20. Koocher G, Keith-Spiegal P. Ethics in psychology. 2nd edition. New York: Oxford University Press; 1998.

21. Rae WA, Brunnquell D, Sullivan JR. Ethical and legal issues in pediatric psychology. In: Roberts MC, editor. Handbook of pediatric psychology. 3rd edition. New York: The Guildford Press; 2003. p. 32–49.

22. Knowles P. Collaborative communication between psychologists and primary care providers. J Clin Psychol Med Settings 2009;16(1):72–6.

23. Walker J, Leveille SG, Ngo L, et al. Inviting patients to read their doctors' notes: patients and doctors look ahead: patient and physician surveys. Ann Intern Med 2011;155(12):811–9.

24. Leveille SG, Walker J, Ralston JD, et al. Evaluating the impact of patients' online access to doctors' visit notes: designing and executing the OpenNotes project. BMC Med Inform Decis Mak 2012;12:32.

25. Walker J, Darer JD, Elmore JG, et al. The road toward fully transparent medical records. N Engl J Med 2014;370(1):6–8.
26. Kahn MW, Bell SK, Walker J, et al. A piece of my mind. Let's show patients their mental health records. JAMA 2014;311(13):1291–2.
27. Wang CJ. Medical documentation in the electronic era. JAMA 2012;308(20): 2091–2.
28. Hanauer DA, Liu Y, Mei Q, et al. Hedging their mets: the use of uncertainty terms in clinical documents and its potential implications when sharing the documents with patients. AMIA Annu Symp Proc 2012;2012:321–30.
29. Blanch DC, Hall JA, Roter DL, et al. Is it good to express uncertainty to a patient? Correlates and consequences for medical students in a standardized patient visit. Patient Educ Couns 2009;76(3):300–6.
30. Ogden J, Fuks K, Gardner M, et al. Doctors expressions of uncertainty and patient confidence. Patient Educ Couns 2002;48(2):171–6.
31. Henry MS. Uncertainty, responsibility, and the evolution of the physician/patient relationship. J Med Ethics 2006;32(6):321–3.
32. Gordon GH, Joos SK, Byrne J. Physician expressions of uncertainty during patient encounters. Patient Educ Couns 2000;40(1):59–65.
33. Kessler RC, Olfson M, Berglund PA. Patterns and predictors of treatment contact after first onset of psychiatric disorders. Am J Psychiatry 1998;155(1):62–9.
34. Tai B, Wu LT, Clark HW. Electronic health records: essential tools in integrating substance abuse treatment with primary care. Subst Abuse Rehabil 2012;3:1–8.
35. Clinical decision support: more than just 'alerts' tipsheet. Centers for Medicare and Medicaid Services; 2014. Available at: https://www.cms.gov/regulations-and-guidance/legislation/EHRincentiveprograms/downloads/clinicaldecisionsupport_tipsheet-.pdf. Accessed June 26, 2016.
36. Romano MJ, Stafford RS. Electronic health records and clinical decision support systems: impact on national ambulatory care quality. Arch Intern Med 2011; 171(10):897–903.
37. Zhou L, Soran CS, Jenter CA, et al. The relationship between electronic health record use and quality of care over time. J Am Med Inform Assoc 2009;16(4): 457–64.
38. Garg AX, Adhikari NK, McDonald H, et al. Effects of computerized clinical decision support systems on practitioner performance and patient outcomes: a systematic review. JAMA 2005;293(10):1223–38.
39. Kaushal R, Shojania KG, Bates DW. Effects of computerized physician order entry and clinical decision support systems on medication safety: a systematic review. Arch Intern Med 2003;163(12):1409–16.
40. Hindahl G. Leading health IT optimization: a next frontier. In: Dewan NA, Luo JS, Lorenzi NM, editors. Mental health practice in a digital world, a clinicians guide. Cham, Switzerland: Springer International Publishing AG; 2015. p. 37–56.
41. Bergman LG, Fors UG. Decision support in psychiatry - a comparison between the diagnostic outcomes using a computerized decision support system versus manual diagnosis. BMC Med Inform Decis Mak 2008;8:9.
42. Rosenman SJ, Korten AE, Levings CT. Computerised diagnosis in acute psychiatry: validity of CIDI-Auto against routine clinical diagnosis. J Psychiatr Res 1997; 31(5):581–92.
43. Lewis G, Sharp D, Bartholomew J, et al. Computerized assessment of common mental disorders in primary care: effect on clinical outcome. Fam Pract 1996; 13:120–6.

44. Cannon DS, Allen SN. A comparison of the effects of computer and manual reminders on compliance with a mental health clinical practice guideline. J Am Med Inform Assoc 2000;7:196–203.

45. Schriger DL, Gibbons PS, Langone CA, et al. Enabling the diagnosis of occult psychiatric illness in the emergency department: a randomized, controlled trial of the computerized, self-administered PRIME-MD diagnostic system. Ann Emerg Med 2001;37:132–40.

46. Rollman BL, Hanusa BH, Lowe HJ, et al. A randomized trial using computerized decision support to improve treatment of major depression in primary care. J Gen Intern Med 2002;17:493–503.

47. Rollman BL, Hanusa BH, Gilbert T, et al. The electronic medical record. A randomized trial of its impact on primary care physicians' initial management of major depression [corrected]. Arch Intern Med 2001;161(2):189–97 [Erratum appears in Arch Intern Med 2001;161(5):705].

48. Duffy FF, Chung H, Trivedi M, et al. Systematic use of patient-rated depression severity monitoring: is it helpful and feasible in clinical psychiatry? Psychiatr Serv 2008;59(10):1148–54.

49. Shelton RC, Trivedi MH. Using algorithms and computerized decision support systems to treat major depression. J Clin Psychiatry 2011;72(12):e36.

50. Trivedi MH, Rush AJ, Crismon ML, et al. Clinical results for patients with major depressive disorder in the Texas Medication Algorithm Project. Arch Gen Psychiatry 2004;61(7):669–80.

51. Trivedi MH, Kern JK, Grannemann BD, et al. A computerized clinical decision support system as a means of implementing depression guidelines. Psychiatr Serv 2004;55(8):879–85.

52. Centers for Disease Control and Prevention. Injury prevention & control: data & statistics (WISQARS). Available at: http://www.cdc.gov/injury/wisqars/leading_causes_death.html. Accessed June 26, 2016.

53. Milton J, Ferguson B, Mills T. Risk assessment and suicide prevention in primary care. Crisis 1999;20(4):171–7.

54. Mane KK, Bizon C, Schmitt C, et al. VisualDecisionLinc: a visual analytics approach for comparative effectiveness-based clinical decision support in psychiatry. J Biomed Inform 2012;45(1):101–6.

55. Horsky J, Schiff GD, Johnston D, et al. Interface design principles for usable decision support: a targeted review of best practices for clinical prescribing interventions. J Biomed Inform 2012;45(6):1202–16.

56. Cifuentes M, Davis M, Fernald D, et al. Electronic health record challenges, workarounds, and solutions observed in practices integrating behavioral health and primary care. J Am Board Fam Med 2015;28(Suppl 1):S63–72.

The Impact of Health Information Technology on the Doctor-Patient Relationship in Child and Adolescent Psychiatry

Rajeev Krishna, MD, PhD

KEYWORDS

- Health information technology • Patient-psychiatrist relationship
- Electronic health records

KEY POINTS

- Health information technology is increasingly permeating psychiatry and behavioral health interactions.
- Limited data suggest that health information technology does not have to negatively impact the patient–provider relationship.
- Thoughtful interaction strategies and appropriate boundary setting strategies are needed to mitigate any potential impacts.

INTRODUCTION

The growth of information technology in health care (health information technology, or HIT) is dramatically altering the landscape in which health care is delivered. For psychiatrists, particularly those operating in larger health systems adopting electronic health records (EHRs), health information technology is now simply a way of life, and the impact on practice must be accounted for. Although HIT creates innumerable new efficiencies and opportunities, it also has significant impact on practice patterns and potentially on the therapeutic relationship, which is of particular relevance to mental health. This article explores the available literature on the impact of HIT on the patient–provider therapeutic relationships across medicine and discusses strategies for managing this impact in the psychiatric relationship.

HOW HEALTH INFORMATION TECHNOLOGY IMPACTS PSYCHIATRIC CARE

The impact of health information technology on the therapeutic relationship between patient and psychiatrist can be felt in several domains. The most obvious is the impact

The author has no conflicts of interest.
Child Psychiatry, Nationwide Children's Hospital, The Ohio State University Wexner Medical Center, 700 Children's Drive, Columbus, OH 43215, USA
E-mail address: Rajeev.Krishna@nationwidechildrens.org

Child Adolesc Psychiatric Clin N Am 26 (2017) 67–75
http://dx.doi.org/10.1016/j.chc.2016.07.007
1056-4993/17/© 2016 Elsevier Inc. All rights reserved.

on the clinical visit itself. The arguably less-intrusive method of pen and paper note taking is increasingly being replaced by a computer monitor and keyboard that demand active attention over the course of the visit and become a third party in the room. Furthermore, the spread of EHRs and the ongoing drive to move psychiatry toward outcome-based care creates opportunities for automated completion and tracking of outcome measures, which can further alter the nature of the visit and the resulting alliance. Although the impact of this new presence has only recently been explored in psychiatry and not at all in child adolescent psychiatry, we may at least fall back on a body of literature from general medicine that has, over the last several decades, explored the effect of electronic health records entering into the medical practice setting.

There are equally concerning but far less well understood effects of recent advances in HIT that warrant consideration. For traditional, office-based providers, the development and propagation of patient portals that allow any patient a direct communication channel to their provider and the expectation of a timely response has clear implications (both positive and negative) on the structure of the therapeutic frame, particularly for patients or families who struggle with appropriate boundaries or may express acute safety concerns through such channels. Indeed, these channels actually provide not just a communication mechanism but an entirely new option for delivering care, as seen by the growth of online care technologies ranging from telehealth efforts such as video-conferenced office visits to email or text/chat-based therapy.

The same HIT infrastructure allowing increased access to providers also raises disclosure and privacy concerns with respect to provider documentation. Patient portals have the capability of providing patients immediate access to their medical records, potentially including immediate access to behavioral health documentation. Although this feature can greatly improve transparency and create new opportunities for therapeutic engagement, it may also greatly disrupt the therapeutic relationship if unexpected and mishandled. This issue is of significant importance given the broad trends toward disclosure of medical records to patients.[1]

The trend of allowing patients access to their medical (and behavioral health) records is preceded only by the trend to allow free access to behavioral health records within a health system, allowing non–behavioral health providers full access to behavioral health documentation and diagnosis. Although this trend greatly expands opportunities to understand and account for mental health illness in general medical decision making, it may also create concerns from patients and families about how to safely discuss concerns with a psychiatrist or mental health specialist while limiting the exposure of important but sensitive topics.

WHAT WE KNOW ABOUT THE EFFECT OF HEALTH INFORMATION TECHNOLOGY ON THE THERAPEUTIC RELATIONSHIP
Electronic Medical Records and the Patient Encounter

There is, unfortunately, little to no hard data on the impact of HIT on the nature of the child and adolescent psychiatry encounter itself. Rather, we must extend from the small knowledge base found in general psychiatry and the larger knowledge base found in general medicine. We must also recognize the high variability in the child and adolescent psychiatry encounter itself. One can reasonably assume that the effects of HIT on interactions with a 17 year-old patient would be different from interactions with a 10-year-old patient. Similarly, interactions with a parent are different from interactions with the child. The differences in these populations compared with adult patients should be kept in mind when considering the available literature. It is also important to note that the available literature generally uses patient satisfaction as a proxy for the quality of the therapeutic relationship.

In assessing the impact of HIT, specifically, EHRs, Stewart and colleagues[2] provide one of the few direct evaluations of HIT in the setting of the psychiatric visit. Their study compares patient satisfaction across numerous domains (based on a modified Patient Satisfaction Questionnaire–Short Form) directly related to the patient–psychiatrist interaction before and after the implementation of an EHR in their psychiatry clinic. They find that, contrary to their own hypothesis, there were no significant changes in patient satisfaction with communication, education, confidentially, anxiety, and several other subscales.[2] Triplett[3] offers a broad review of the literature on the effect of EHRs in psychiatric practice, making note of the importance of the narrative to the field and raising the question of how much this narrative interpretation may be lost both in time spent interacting with an EHR and in the tendency to follow a more scripted interview style based on EHR prompts. Although the article by Triplett[3] focuses on the overall impact of the EHR, such changes to communication patterns affect not only the quality of evaluation, but the relationship itself.[3] Rasminsky and colleagues[4] raise this same point in a commentary describing a case scenario in which a resident, attending more to the EHR than to the patient's affect, missed the key affective reactions that revealed the patient's true underlying condition.

Extending into the relevant literature in general medicine, there is support both for the general observation that HIT has minimal impact on patient satisfaction and on the patient–physician relationship and for the specific concerns that may most impact a psychiatric practice. The general medical literature over the last 20 years consistently shows that computers in the examining room do not have a negative effect on patient perceptions of the encounter or the physician and may even increase patient satisfaction.[5–9] Broadly, the underlying theme in these studies is that computers have become so common that their use during a medical visit is unremarkable. In some instances, communication actually improved with the introduction of an EHR.[10] Underlying this broadly neutral trend, however, are certain characteristics that are potentially concerning to psychiatry. Makoul and colleagues[11] make note that physicians using an EHR produced more complete assessments but note a trend of physicians using the EHR to have less focus on psychosocial issues or issues of how illness affects a patient's life when compared with control physicians without an EHR. Similarly, McGrath and colleagues,[12] in a small study, found that physician interaction with an EHR can alter or disrupt nonverbal communication between physician and patient, which can alter rapport building, patient comfort, and disclosure patterns.[13] Of notable concern in this collection of data is that these components of a medical encounter (psychosocial assessments, evaluation and monitoring of nonverbal communication patterns, and careful rapport building), although sometimes ancillary to a general medical visit, actually form much of the core of the psychiatric assessment, particularly in more therapy-oriented modalities. As such, the effect of an EHR may be notably greater than in a general medical practice setting.

Internet Technologies and Online Communication

Although EHRs may have the greatest direct impact or patient–provider interactions given their place at the center of the psychiatric encounter, the actual adoption of EHRs in psychiatry has been slow.[14] As such, some of the first interactions of many solo practitioners with health information technology may be through electronic communication mechanisms. It is no longer odd for even a traditional office-based provider to engage with patients or families over email, patient portals, and other electronic media, offering therapeutic direction and recommendations. This section focuses on the impact of such communication forms on the therapeutic relationship specifically.

Although there is some literature on the use of patient portals as a patient education medium, no studies seem to exist on the impact of patient portals on the patient–provider relationship in the mental health field. The limited data in medicine as a whole generally recognizes patient portals as leading to an overall increase in patient satisfaction,[15] although some literature suggests that actual use of patient portals does, in fact, relate inversely to the quality of the doctor-patient relationship (ie, patients turn more to portals when they feel the ability to communicate directly is inadequate).[16]

Although the data on patient portals in particular in limited, a growing body of evidence exists in the adult literature on the formation of therapeutic relationships in treatment modalities that are entirely online (eg, telehealth, chat/email therapy). Recent review articles note that the available literature is scant but suggest that aspects of the therapeutic relationship in such online treatment modalities may be comparable to face-to-face visits.[17,18] These studies primarily explore therapy delivered online (as opposed to medication management) and draw from adult populations directly receiving treatment (as opposed to child populations or parents).

Privacy of Behavioral Health Records

The literature offers no information on the impact of expanding access to behavioral health records to other disciplines on the patient–provider relationship within psychiatry itself (for example, with patients less willing to discuss issues with the psychiatrist or other providers raising sensitive issues inappropriately and thus breaking patient confidence in the psychiatrist). Anecdotally, the authors worked at several institutions where routine mental health visit documentation is freely available to other disciplines within the health system, and the impact on patient/provider interaction overall is thought to be minimal. This impact ultimately must be evaluated on a case by case basis.

MANAGING HEALTH INFORMATION TECHNOLOGY CONCERNS IN PSYCHIATRIC PRACTICE
Electronic Health Records and the Psychiatric Encounter

Although the available literature suggests a minimal impact of EHRs on the physician–patient relationship in general medicine[5–9] and in general psychiatry,[2] it also suggests changes to the quality of assessment, rapport building, and monitoring of effect.[11–13] This literature, although not directly speaking to child psychiatry, offers strategies for mitigating the most harmful potential effects of EHRs on the therapeutic encounter. The following should be considered when using an EHR during a child psychiatry encounter.

Excessive attention to the computer

Although data suggest patients are tolerant of computer use during the encounter, psychiatric visits involve collecting and documenting a far greater narrative component and could lead to greater overall disengagement from the patient. Several simple steps can help mitigate this:

- Review the patient's chart before the visit allowing for immediate engagement with the patient rather than an initial chart review.
- Learn/practice touch typing, allowing narrative data entry while maintaining direct contact with the patient and family.

- Defer extensive data entry (longer periods of typing or dictation) until after the visit.
- Set aside time during the visit to disengage from the computer and focus full attention on the patient and family.
- Similarly, set aside time for completing work on the computer. Talk to patients and families about what you are doing on the EHR to maintain engagement. Data from medical visits suggest that patients will be highly tolerant of computer use during medical portions of the visit such as medication review or prescription entry.

Eye contact/missed affect or nonverbal cues

Data from the existing literature suggests that, regardless of actual patient satisfaction, an EHR does change patient–provider communication patterns. This finding is particularly relevant in psychiatry. Consider the following strategies to mitigate this effect:

- Office arrangement: if possible, arrange the office space so that the computer can be operated while facing the patient/family, avoiding arrangements that place the computer physically between provider and patient. This arrangement maximizes opportunities to monitor affect and nonverbal cues even while attending to the EHR.
- Recognize that eye contact is a potential problem area and make explicit effort to maintain awareness of patient affect and level of engagement. Be prepared to defer documentation and fully focus on the patient and family if EHR use seems to be leading to disengagement.

Online Communication

As noted, there are relatively little formal data available discussing the impact of online communication mechanisms on the therapeutic alliance, although broadly speaking, such mechanisms do seem to improve patient satisfaction.[15] The existence of entirely online therapeutic modalities and the data suggesting a comparable therapeutic alliance compared with face-to-face visits[17,18] should provide reassurance for those providers who make use of online communication methodologies to augment their office visits and for those providers who participate in telehealth and other online care modalities in general.

ONLINE PATIENT–PROVIDER COMMUNICATION

Ultimately, as a communication medium, patient portals, emails, and other technology-driven systems are conceptually similar to telephones, voice mails, letters, and other forms of outside-of-visit patient–provider communication that mental health professionals have dealt with for decades. As such, in the context of augmenting office-based visits with online communication, it can be argued that the existing collective knowledge in managing patient communication, boundary setting, and therapeutic alliance may be applied. Several nuances of online communication should be considered and discussed with patients before engaging in online communication:

Privacy

E-mail, online chat, short message service (SMS) messaging, and many other forms of network-based communication are not inherently secure for communicating protected health information. In practice, many patients and parents prefer the convenience of direct exchanges over the protection of secure portals; however, the options that a provider is willing to make available and the risks should be discussed, agreed on, and documented before online communication begins. This communication will help clarify and define the boundaries of the treatment relationship and minimize later miscommunication. In approaching this, providers may consider the following points to protect both themselves and their patients:

- The Health Insurance Portability and Accountability Act (HIPAA) does not prohibit plain text E-mail exchanges with patients; however, there is an expectation that reasonable safeguards are taken to ensure the correct recipient and to ensure that patients are willing to communicate by this mechanism and understand the risks.[19]
- Although HIPAA does not prohibit text messaging, the use of standard SMS messages (as opposed to more secure instant messaging options that are available) is problematic from several technical and security dimensions and should not be undertaken without full understanding of these nuances.[20]

Reliability

Although secure messaging systems generally maintain an audit trail, the reliability of most forms of Internet communication cannot be guaranteed. There is frequently also an expectation of more rapid response to such communication than a provider may actually offer. Expected response time and reliable backup communication options should be discussed as part of defining communication parameters.

ONLINE CARE DELIVERY

Providers of telehealth and other online care modalities have a different set of challenges with respect to the therapeutic relationship. Although available data suggest that a comparable relationship to face-to-face communication can be achieved,[17,18] in practice this is probably most true of interactions with parents as opposed to pediatric patients. Creating engagement with a disruptive child or a depressed and inherently disengaged teenager over a video display presents unique challenges for which the current literature does not account. By contrast, texting or other online communication strategies may actually achieve better engagement with the same disengaged teenager than even a face-to-face visit might achieve. Ultimately, the strategy for negotiating these nuances must account for an individual provider's practice patterns and comfort with technology. Although the aforementioned concerns of privacy and reliability remain as true with online care delivery, there are further considerations that might be made.

Face-to-Face Visits

Recognizing that face-to-face may not be practical for certain practice patterns, efforts to maintain some frequency of such visits (eg, initial visit or once per year) can be valuable to ground the therapeutic alliance. Experience with initial face-to-face visits and telehealth follow-up suggest that this model can be effective for establishing a relationship that can subsequently be maintained over electronic communication.

Personal Versus Professional Communication

Many of the alternative online communication infrastructures available may also be used regularly by providers as part of their personal communications and interactions (eg, text messaging, social media). Providers should set up separate accounts for business and personal use whenever possible and to be highly aware of the causal boundary violations that can easily occur through such informal communication infrastructures. These violations could range from inadvertently sending a personal text message to a patient to intentionally divulging excessive personal information or breaking the nature of the therapeutic relationship in other ways because the personal distance created by the communication media inherently reduces some of the social barriers to such boundary violations.

Behavioral Health Documentation

A final consideration on the impact of HIT is the effect of broader access to provider documentation. Specific concerns are the impact of patients and families having access to provider documentation without opportunities for providers to discuss the meaning of formulations and the impact of other health care professionals reviewing mental health charts and either discussing sensitive issues with patients (disrupting trust in the relationship with the mental health provider) or altering care based on a poor understanding of certain psychiatric diagnosis (borderline or cluster B traits). Although the effects of these concerns cannot currently be quantified, the following considerations may aid in managing the therapeutic relationship in these situations.

Early discussion

Because confidentiality should be discussed with patients and families as part of the initial encounter, so too should the potential scope of access to their health records. Strategies for discussing sensitive topics while maintaining the patient's desired level of confidentiality should be agreed on up front.

Limit speculation

Documentation of speculative formulations should be limited, particularly those that may carry negative connotations when reviewed by other providers or by patients themselves. Although behavioral health records are often afforded a higher level of protection from release without provider approval than many other medical records, it should be assumed when documenting that a patient may read their records without a prior discussion opportunity.

Early transparency

Whenever possible or not clinically contraindicated, providers should be upfront with patients and families about the formulation and diagnosis that will be entered into the medical record. This may not only avoid later problems with disclosures but may create new avenues for discussing sensitive or difficult topics.

SUMMARY

Health information technology has the potential to revolutionize care delivery in many ways. The particular value of the therapeutic relationship in psychiatry makes the potential of HIT to affect this relationship alarming. Although limited, the available literature fortunately suggests that HIT has many positive effects and may have only specific negative effects on the therapeutic relationship that can be mitigated with simple practices and thoughtful clinical skill and judgment. For the child and adolescent psychiatrist, the available literature may offer the greatest insight into the impact of HIT or interactions with parents and older patients. The common theme, however, remains a focus on maintaining active engagement with patients and families to capture those critical moments of affect and nonverbal communication that often reveal underlying truths and building the rapport needed to bring those hidden truths to light. Ensuring that HIT remains an augmentation to this process and not a replacement for it will be the key to making these new technologies a valuable part of the therapeutic relationship.

REFERENCES

1. Ricciardi L. Building momentum: expanding patient access to medical records - health IT buzz. health IT buzz. Office of the National Coordinator for Health Information Technology. 2013. Available at: https://www.healthit.gov/buzz-blog/consumer/building-momentum-expanding-patient-access-medical-records/. Accessed July 4, 2016.
2. Stewart RF, Kroth PJ, Schuyler M, et al. Do electronic health records affect the patient-psychiatrist relationship? A before & after study of psychiatric outpatients. BMC Psychiatry 2010;10(1):3.
3. Triplett P. Psychiatry and the meaningful use of electronic health records. Perspect Biol Med 2013;56(3):407–21.
4. Rasminsky S, Berman R, Burt VK. Are we turning our backs on our patients? Training psychiatrists in the era of the electronic health record. Am J Psychiatry AJP 2015;172(8):708–9.
5. Aydin CE, Rosen PN, Jewell SM, et al. Computers in the examining room: the patient's perspective. Proc Annu Symp Comput Appl Med Care 1995;824.
6. Koide D, Asonuma M, Naito K, et al. Evaluation of electronic health records from viewpoint of patients. Stud Health Technol Inform 2006;122:304.
7. Ridsdale L, Hudd S. Computers in the consultation: the patient's view. Br J Gen Pract 1994;44(385):367–9.
8. Garrison GM, Bernard ME, Rasmussen NH. 21st-century health care: the effect of computer use by physicians on patient satisfaction at a family medicine clinic. Fam Med 2002;34(5):362–8.
9. Delpierre C. A systematic review of computer-based patient record systems and quality of care: more randomized clinical trials or a broader approach? Int J Qual Health Care 2004;16(5):407–16.
10. Johnson KB, Serwint JR, Fagan LA, et al. Computer-based documentation: effects on parent-provider communication during pediatric health maintenance encounters. Pediatrics 2008;122(3):590–8.
11. Makoul G, Curry RH, Tang PC. The use of electronic medical records: communication patterns in outpatient encounters. J Am Med Inform Assoc 2001;8(6):610–5.
12. Mcgrath JM, Arar NH, Pugh JA. The influence of electronic medical record usage on nonverbal communication in the medical interview. Health Informatics J 2007; 13(2):105–18.
13. Duggan P, Parrott L. Physicians' nonverbal rapport building and patients' talk about the subjective component of illness. Hum Commun Res Hum Comm Res 2001;27(2):299–311.
14. Kokkonen EW, Davis SA, Lin HC, et al. Use of electronic medical records differs by specialty and office settings. J Am Med Inform Assoc 2013;20(e1):e33–8.
15. Lin C-T, Wittevrongel L, Moore L, et al. An internet-based patient-provider communication system: randomized controlled trial. J Med Internet Res J Med Internet Res 2005;7(4):e47.
16. Zickmund SL, Hess R, Bryce CL, et al. Interest in the use of computerized patient portals: role of the provider–patient relationship. J Gen Intern Med 2007;23(S1):20–6.
17. Sucala M, Schnur JB, Constantino MJ, et al. The therapeutic relationship in e-therapy for mental health: a systematic review. J Med Internet Res J Med Internet Res 2012; 14(4):e110.

18. Berger T. The therapeutic alliance in internet interventions: a narrative review and suggestions for future research. Psychotherapy Res 2016;1–14.
19. Does the HIPAA privacy rule permit health care providers to use e-mail to discuss health issues and treatment with their patients? Heath Information Privacy - Frequently Asked Questions. US Department of Health and Human Services. 2008. Available at: http://www.hhs.gov/hipaa/for-professionals/faq/570/does-hipaa-permit-health-care-providers-to-use-email-to-discuss-health-issues-with-patients/. Accessed July 5, 2016.
20. Lakhani A. "HIPAA-COMPLIANT" Texting of PHI: The Good. The Bad. The Ugly. TechHealth Perspectives. 2013. Available at: http://www.techhealthperspectives.com/2013/10/14/hipaa-compliant-texting-of-phi/. Accessed July 15, 2015.

Considerations for Conducting Telemental Health with Children and Adolescents

Eve-Lynn Nelson, PhD[a,b],*, Sharon Cain, MD[c], Susan Sharp, DO[c]

KEYWORDS

- Telemental health • Telemedicine • Telepsychiatry • Health information technologies
- Outreach with underserved populations

KEY POINTS

- Child and adolescent telemental health has been practiced successfully across underserved settings with diverse youth, for most psychiatric disorders, and across development.
- Assessment and treatments have been provided successfully using secure videoconferencing, including pharmacotherapy and psychotherapy.
- Although evidence is emerging concerning the efficacy of telemental health, care should adhere to evidence-based guidelines and best practices set forth by professional organizations.
- Across telemental health clinic start up and implementation, close attention should be given to administrative issues, legal/regulatory considerations (eg, licensure, credentialing, reimbursement, prescribing regulations), and technical support at the teleprovider and patient sites.

INTRODUCTION

Child mental health disorders are an important public health issue in the United States because of their prevalence, early onset, and impact on the child, family, and community, with an estimated total annual cost of $247 billion. Approximately 20% of children

Drs E.-L. Nelson and S. Sharp have nothing to disclose. Dr S. Cain participates in clinical research at the University of Kansas in collaboration with Duke University for a study sponsored by Pfizer Pharmaceutical. This research is unrelated to the current article.
[a] Pediatrics Department, University of Kansas Medical Center, 3901 Rainbow Boulevard, Kansas City, KS 66160, USA; [b] KU Center for Telemedicine and Telehealth, University of Kansas Medical Center, 4330 Shawnee Mission Parkway, Suite 136, MS 7001, Fairway, KS 66205, USA; [c] Psychiatry & Behavioral Sciences Department, University of Kansas Medical Center, MS 4015, 3901 Rainbow Boulevard, Kansas City, KS 66160, USA
* Corresponding author. KU Center for Telemedicine and Telehealth, University of Kansas Medical Center, 4330 Shawnee Mission Parkway, Suite 136, Mail Stop 7001, Fairway, KS 66205.
E-mail address: enelson2@kumc.edu

living in the United States experience a mental disorder in a given year, and surveillance during 1994 to 2011 has shown the prevalence of these conditions to be increasing.[1] Despite recent initiatives designed to expand behavioral health services for youth, such as the Patient Protection and Affordable Care Act, many children in need of mental health care still do not receive it, receive an inadequate "dose" of sessions, or receive services from local providers without specialty training with children or without training in evidence-based pediatric approaches. Even greater health disparities are seen across geographies and ethnicities.[2]

As part of telemedicine clinical services, telemental health offers an innovative way to address striking access gaps. The umbrella term refers to behavioral and mental health services that are provided via synchronous telecommunications technologies, including discipline-specific applications such as telepsychiatry and telepsychology.[3] Secure videoconferencing technology allows providers and patients/families at different locations to interact in real time and strives to ensure comparable treatment to traditional face-to-face settings. It is a relatively low-cost technology solution because behavioral health interventions largely rely on verbal communication and observation rather than the need for more expensive peripheral devices.[4]

Because youth often have a comfort level and extensive exposure to technologies, telemedicine may be a particularly good fit for this age group. Telemental health saves telemental health providers, or teleproviders, the time and expense of travel and has been extended to both rural and urban settings.[4] There are additional benefits of this telemedicine approach in connecting systems of care and enhancing care coordination. Supervised settings that include a telepresenter, such as clinics, hospitals, primary care practices, schools, daycare facilities, detention centers, and other settings, have been the most frequent sites of connection with youth and have been associated with reimbursement. Unsupervised settings such as homes are increasingly being considered with the expansion of secure videoconferencing over mobile devices. The authors summarize telemental health basics around the *why*, *what*, *when*, *where*, *who*, and *how* associated with safe and effective care.

WHY DELIVER CHILD TELEMENTAL HEALTH SERVICES?

Telemental health expansion is driven by increasing expectations for high-quality behavioral health services across geographies. Telemental health is further advanced by the decreasing cost of secure videoconferencing options and increasing access to high-speed connectivity. Health care reform has increased interest in creative solutions to increase access to behavioral health services due to access challenges associated with the shortages of youth behavioral health specialists, a maldistribution of available specialists, a shrinking behavioral health specialist workforce, and instability in behavioral health funding.[5] Rural and frontier communities are particularly hard hit with access difficulties because of shrinking populations, declining economies, and increasing poverty as well as delays in treatment, less access to mental health insurance, and limited transportation options.[6,7] The burdens of traveling for services are often magnified, with the frequent standard of care for regular sessions sustained over a period of time.

Patients and families report several reasons for participating in telemental health, and as with most telemedicine specialties, report high satisfaction with telemental health.[8] These reasons include the following:

1. Conveniently finding high-quality services close to home;
2. Decreasing time away from both work and school;
3. Decreasing costs associated with traveling miles for care;

4. Decreasing stresses of travel with a child with a behavior disorder and siblings;
5. Decreasing worries about navigating unfamiliar health care settings;
6. Allowing additional supporters to attend and work together to coordinate care; and
7. Decreasing stigma by connecting to child friendly settings such as schools.

For some patients and families, videoconferencing offers advantages, including less self-consciousness, increased personal space especially for adolescents,[9] and decreased confidentiality concerns as the teleprovider is outside of the local community.

WHAT CONSTITUTES TELEMENTAL HEALTH?

A first consideration in what is meant by telemental health relates to the model of service delivery. Several telemental health models have been used to provide services to youth, each with a slightly different purpose.[4] Telemental health services directly provided to the patient/family in supervised settings has been the most common service delivery model with youth and is the focus of this article. Other models complement these efforts, including consultation models that use videoconferencing to link the behavioral health specialist with the local PCP, supporting "virtual curbside consultation." In addition, workforce capacity building models use videoconferencing to blend telehealth and distance education. Pioneered at the University of New Mexico, the Extension of Community Healthcare Outcomes (ECHO) model uses secure videoconferencing technology to connect multiple health care providers to a multidisciplinary team around a range of behavioral health topics (eg, attention-deficit/hyperactivity disorder [ADHD], autism, substance abuse intervention). The telementoring approach pairs weekly brief didactic updates around best practices with deidentified case presentations from the participating sites in order to build a community of practice. ECHO promotes increasing medical home and rural primary care collaboration with specialists and reducing variation in care using clinical best practices and algorithms.[10] Some programs have developed specific models for consultation to primary care,[11,12] including one that moves flexibly between consultation and direct care.[13]

In describing the "what," or the content of telemental health services, comprehensive literature reviews inform the content of telemental health with children and adolescents.[4,8] Because of the small but emerging child literature, lessons are often drawn as a downward extension from adult literature.[14] Bashshur and colleagues[15] completed a recent review of the empirical literature for telemental heath across the lifespan following rigorous inclusion criteria. Overall, they concluded that there is strong and consistent evidence of the feasibility of telemental health as well as high acceptability across teleproviders and patients. Based on rating of the highest quality of scientific design, there was indication of improvement in symptoms and quality of life among patients across a broad range of demographic and diagnostic groups.

Although the literature base is small, comprehensive reviews of the child telemental health overall[4,8,16] reflect good outcomes across child behavioral presenting concerns, in both rural and urban settings. Findings reflect adequate diagnostic efficacy, feasibility, and satisfaction across patients, families, teleproviders, and referring physicians.

With large sample sizes, 3 studies provide guidance specific to telepharmacotherapy with children and adolescents. Two retrospective chart reviews describe the results of telepsychiatry consultation. One study[17] reviewed the charts of 223 patients and found that consultation resulted in changes in diagnosis (48%), treatment (81.6%), and clinical improvement (60.1%). In the second study, 100 patient charts were reviewed after consultation. The results showed that consultation was associated with changes in diagnosis and treatment. Twenty-seven percent of those recommendations involved starting or managing medication, including stimulants, antidepressants, and antipsychotics.[18]

There is only one randomized trial noted specific to pediatric pharmacologic treatment with children.[19] Myers and colleagues[19] randomized 233 children diagnosed with ADHD to receive 22 weeks of treatment in 1 of 2 groups. The active control group received a single telepsychiatry consultation, with recommendations made to primary care providers (PCPs) to implement at their discretion during the trial. The intervention group received 6 sessions of pharmacotherapy via videoconferencing during the 22-week trial, complemented by caregiver behavior training delivered in person by a community therapist who was trained and supervised remotely. Findings suggest that the telepsychiatrists demonstrated high fidelity to consensus-based pharmacotherapy algorithms. Participants in both the intervention and the consultation groups improved, and those who received the 6-session intervention showed significantly better ADHD outcomes per caregivers' reports than did the consultation group. In addition, the caregivers themselves reported improved functioning.[20] This study provides high-quality evidence for the ability to provide guideline-based care through videoconferencing and the "added value" that a short-term telepsychiatric intervention provides over a single teleconsultation to primary care.

There are also a handful of studies focused on child clinical interventions using videoconferencing.[21,22] Lessons may be drawn from the more robust adult therapy literature, with roughly equivalent clinical outcomes using evidence-based practices to treat posttraumatic stress disorder, depression and anxiety, eating disorders, and substance abuse concerns and similar process findings across therapy satisfaction, alliance, attendance, and completion.[23] Individual therapy using videoconferencing has also been successfully implemented with urban and rural children in a variety of settings, with reports most often using cognitive-behavioral approaches.[24] Most studies have been therapy interventions for ADHD, but there are also examples in autism, behavioral concerns with juvenile offenders, depression, obsessive compulsive disorder, and tic disorders.[3,21]

Telemental health has been shown effective with behavioral health interventions to support chronic illnesses.[21] Case reports suggest the delivery can be used for supportive interventions with children with a range of conditions (eg, cancer, congenital heart disease, cystic fibrosis, diabetes, epilepsy, irritable bowel disorder) and their caregivers. In addition, an emerging literature suggests effectiveness of individual and group interventions to treat pediatric obesity.[25]

WHEN IS A TELEPROVIDER READY TO BEGIN SERVICE?

Motivated to increase access for very needed behavioral health services, teleproviders and health systems are often drawn to the technology's potential and eager to begin services quickly. As with implementing any new onsite outreach service, it is advisable to consider a 12- to 18-month start-up period in order to ensure the safest care for the patients following ethical, legal, and regulatory best practices. This period allows relationship building with community sites to consider the long-term business planning and sustainability[26] from both the teleprovider and the patient sites, including administrative (eg, scheduling, billing), technical support, and legal/regulatory needs.

Establishing a Telemental Health Service

Technology makes it possible for teleproviders to offer services across the city, the state, the country, or even the world in real time. There is high need across settings so it is important to take a thoughtful approach to timeframe and site selection. The developmental model of Shore and Manson[27] for rural telepsychiatry guides overall considerations in starting a child telemental health practice. They emphasize that the telemental health clinic purpose drives technology selection. It is sometimes difficult to avoid the marketing buzz for the newest technologies, which may or may not be a fit for the telemental health. A comprehensive *Needs Assessment* informs what telemental health services are of highest need/interest. The teleprovider has ongoing discussion across stakeholders, including community leaders, community organizations, consumer groups, local behavioral and mental health providers, local PCPs, and other key partners. A detailed assessment of the existing technological, organizational, and programmatic infrastructure at the outreach site or sites as well as within the teleprovider's own organization is recommended, including the equipment available and/or needed; the clinical space; the connectivity available (as well as the overall networking burden of the televideo application); the expectations concerning who will pay for equipment/connectivity over time; and staffing needs.

In addition, new telemental health services should clearly define roles and responsibilities across parties through clear protocols, including careful consideration of budget requirements immediately and long term, and reimbursement option for the target population.[28] About half of states have telemedicine parity, meaning that if services are reimbursed by the insurer in onsite settings then they are also reimbursed over telemedicine; this helps teleproviders and families consistently know what telemental health services will be reimbursed.[29] A Pilot Implementation phase, focused on a small-scale trial and continuous improvement, can assist in refining processes and promoting sustainability.

Ethical and Regulatory Considerations

The careful consideration and planning around regulatory and ethical issues also impact when the telemental health program may launch. Just as in on-site clinical settings, the core ethical concern to protect the patient remains paramount for videoconferencing settings.[5,21] In addition, professional guidelines addressing telemental health are emerging to inform "reasonable steps" for telemental health practice across clinical, administrative, and technical considerations, including child-specific guidelines.[30] Telemental health guidelines include the American Academy of Child and Adolescent Psychiatry,[31] the American Psychological Association,[32] as well as a growing list of other organizations.[3] Existing guidelines from the American Telemedicine Association[33,34] as well as soon to be released child telemental health guidelines and general pediatric practice guidelines are excellent resources.

At the national level, The Joint Commission for the Accreditation of Healthcare Organizations has regulations applicable to telemedicine. Federal, state, and local laws, as well as institutional requirements, must also be reviewed related to the following: (1) involuntary commitment and reporting child maltreatment; (2) teleprovider credentialing and privileging requirements; and (3) malpractice insurance specific to telemedicine.[35]

Interstate licensure is a complex issue; the teleprovider is encouraged to review state licensure requirements related to the teleprovider location and the patient location. In most states, the teleprovider is required to hold a license where the patient is being seen; some states have additional requirements. Other regulatory/ethical requirements to consider include verifying the patient identity and confirming the location of the patient[34]; this is often more easily accomplished in supervised than in unsupervised settings/homes. It is equally important for the teleprovider to inform the patient of the teleprovider's location and credentials.

Other important factors to consider when initiating a telemental health service include the patient's privacy and compliance of the videoconferencing transmission with the Health Insurance Portability and Accountability Act. State law regarding confidentiality of behavioral health information should be reviewed, and when applicable, school-specific confidentiality requirements as outlined in the Family Educational Rights and Privacy Act Regulations. Informed consent for treatment may include an additional consent to receive telemental health services. A review of the potential limitations and acknowledgment of the patients' right to refuse treatment over videoconferencing is part of informed consent as well as clarification of whether the sessions will be recorded and/or stored in any way. Best practices in documentation and use of the electronic health record should also be followed.

WHERE ARE PATIENTS AND FAMILIES RECEIVING TELEMENTAL HEALTH SERVICES?

In order to increase access for children and families, there has been much creativity in "meeting the child and family where they're at" and deliver services as conveniently as possible. Direct-to-consumer telemental health vendors and private practice teleproviders are expanding delivery sites. It is important to keep in mind the unique needs across settings and carefully consider the ethical, regulatory, and training needs as later discussed in the "how" section.

Supervised settings are the most frequently reported sites of youth telemental health services, including rural and urban settings. Examples include schools, outpatient clinics, primary care clinics, community mental health centers, physician offices, and correctional settings.[36] Individual reports describe delivery to other settings such as residential treatment facilities, critical access hospitals, group homes, Area Health Education Centers, colleges, sites serving foster care, military bases, inpatient psychiatry settings, and daycare centers.[5,22] Unsupervised settings including patient homes are emerging points of service delivery that bring both new benefits and risks[3] due to decreased teleprovider control over the environment.

With a focus on family-centered assessment and treatment, telemental health services are being moved outside of traditional mental health care settings. These settings offer advantages in identifying contextual factors involved in youths' behavior and mental health needs as well as in working with a wide range of caregivers/supporters involved in implementing recommendations. One collaborative opportunity is using the technology to link teleproviders with PCPs. Telemental health affords increased communication and coordination to benefit the child and family, support positive outcomes,[37] and has the potential to advance patient-centered medical home ideals.[38]

In addition, school-based telemental health services engage youth during the school day, thereby reducing missed school days, decreasing disruption in the child's classroom time and parent's workday, allowing parents to be involved in a setting that is familiar and convenient, and incorporating school personnel into treatment planning.[39] In addition to direct telemental health services, the technology allows the youth's teleproviders to engage in multidisciplinary planning, student evaluation, Individualized Education Plan/504 plan meetings, and collaboration with teachers, school specialists (eg, school psychologists, social workers, and allied health specialists), nurses, and administrators.[33] Distance education for staff around behavioral health topics as well as consultation on both classroom-specific and general school issues, provides unique opportunities to support children and adolescents and deliver guideline-adherent care.[40]

Residential treatment centers and correctional settings often require prolonged separations between the confined youth and their family and local providers.[5,41] Although privacy and confidentiality must be carefully considered, telemental health allows families to participate in a youth's treatment while remaining in their home communities or allow a teleprovider to connect to the youth's facility. Home-based telemental health offers potential advantages to observe the youth in a naturalistic setting and to practice skills in the lived environment. Comer and colleagues[42] are pioneering the evaluation of delivering telemental health interventions for early onset behavior disorders delivered to the home. A recent feasibility study[43] successfully delivered home-based telemental health services to children who had experienced trauma and found that trauma-informed care elements could be translated to the home-based setting. Finally, positive results are emerging from a nationwide clinical trial across the lifespan that evaluated support group services for homebound individuals and their caregivers using mobile tablets for videoconferencing. Early reports[44] note positive, cost-effective results related to satisfaction and health outcomes.

WHO PARTICIPATES IN TELEMENTAL HEALTH SERVICES?

This section addresses the different people involved in telemental health encounters, including the patient and family, the therapist and trainees, the telepresenter (in supervised settings), and the community stakeholders/supporters.

Patients and Family

Across telemental health clinics, patients tend to present with the same concerns as seen in traditional clinic settings.[33] No presentation or diagnostic category has been excluded from telemental health services. However, the same careful consideration used in traditional clinics is taken related to competence with the presenting concern as well as access to requisite resources, particularly with severely impaired patients. The choice of who will be seen depends on developmental and diagnostic considerations, personnel and resources at the distant site, patient and guardian preferences, the teleprovider's judgment, and input from the referring provider.[31] The teleprovider should make sure there are appropriate on-site clinical resources in order to safely conduct an evaluation, including resources to support patients in crisis. Depending on the situation, exclusion criteria may include factors such as youth without accompanying guardians, patients without a PCP, or patients with a PCP who are uncomfortable resuming care for psychiatric patients. Unsupervised setting may have additional inclusion/exclusion considerations in order to ensure patient safety. For example, the report of a current or previous person in the home who as acted violently and abusively may be contraindicated due to concerns the person could be off screen and able to eavesdrop, or may become violent or impulsively disconnect during a session.[3,43]

Teleproviders and Their Trainees

There is no profile distinguishing between teleproviders who choose to engage in telemental health, although it is not uncommon that they also engage in onsite outreach and value a community. Common goals noted by teleproviders include the following:

- Strive to translate the same effective communication and intervention skills that they use in the onsite setting to the telemedicine context;
- Provide services within the scope of their appropriate practice for in person encounters, including the necessary education, training, cultural competency, and ongoing continuing education/professional development; and
- Set appropriate expectations regarding the telehealth encounter, including, for example, prescribing policies, scope of service, communication, and follow-up. Familiarizing oneself with the federal Controlled Substances Act (US Code Title 21) and other relevant state and federal regulations is important.

Because of the newness of the field, there are no established performance competencies specific to technology, but telehealth guidelines provide direction.[31,33] Hilty and colleagues[45] have proposed an innovative competency model aligning telemental health competencies with the Accreditation Council for Graduate Medical Education framework. These telemental health competencies span patient care, system- and practice-based learning, professionalism, communication, knowledge, and technology. The competencies encompass novice or advanced beginner, competent/proficient, and expert levels. Following adult learning best practices, teaching and assessment methods for the telemental health competencies are outlined. Additional resources are available through both the federally funded telehealth resource centers (www.telehealthresourcecenter.org) and public and private programs (eg, www.tmhguide.org, others).

Teleproviders need practice with the technology as well as cultural competence with the population served and communication skills in working across systems of care. Ideally, new teleproviders shadow and receive guidance from established teleproviders and complete "test" runs in order to build confidence with the technology. Federally funded telehealth resource centers, professional organizations such as the American Telemedicine Association, and training companies offer training related to these competencies.[3]

It is appealing to include trainees in telemental health clinics in order to encourage consideration of future outreach practice and the rewards of working with underserved children and their families across systems of care. Training resource and supervision should be considered as well as opportunities for trainees to engage in telemental health evaluation efforts. Telemental health offers unique training advantages because several trainees can be unobtrusive in the telemedicine room without crowding the patient.[46,47]

Telepresenter

The telepresenter, sometimes called a presenter or facilitator, at the distant site facilitates sessions and is often the site's "champion." This telepresenter is someone with a clinical background trained in the use of videoconferencing equipment to "present" the patient and manage the technical components of the encounter[48]; additional training around supporting behavioral health patients may also be beneficial. The telepresenter serves as the bridge between the therapist and the patient/family at the distant site and assists by promoting the telemental health service, scheduling the consult, compiling intake packets, socializing the patient/family to televideo, using the technology, assisting during the consultation, and helping the patient/family follow-up on recommendations. Thus, the telepresenter requires support across administrative leaders and colleagues in completing these many tasks as they may be in addition to typical responsibilities and workflow.

Multiple Informants

Videoconferencing often links together systems of care by connecting the teleprovider with schools, rural clinics, primary care offices, and other systems. Increased communication across technology systems represented by these multiple informants is a chief advantage of telemental health. If the patient is under the age of 18, the parent/guardian guides who participates in sessions, but generally welcomes these additional support personnel in developing and implementing the treatment plan. The videoconferencing session allows everyone to contribute their unique piece to the diagnostic and treatment puzzle. Communication occurs not only with the teleprovider but also with each other. For example, it is a frequent situation in school-based clinics that parents and teachers have had very little or no direct communication about the child's behavior in different settings or family stressors that may be impacting the child's functioning.

HOW IS CHILD TELEMENTAL HEALTH IMPLEMENTED?

The authors first describe overarching elements that relate to quality of care in telemental health practice.[3–5] They then summarize specific considerations related to evaluation and pharmacology. One overarching consideration is support for diverse families, including resources for interpreting needs, needs around hearing impairment, mobility needs in accessing the telemental health space, and other culture- and community-specific considerations.

Confidential Clinical Space at the Patient and Teleprovider Sites

An ideal room is large enough to accommodate the youth, a clinical staff person, and at least 2 other adults, but not so large that it encourages distractibility or hyperactivity. The room should be large enough to evaluate children's motor skills, play, and exploration and to note abnormal movements.[4] A table allows the child to draw or play but should not interfere with viewing motor skills. Some developmental teams prefer not to have tables in the room to decrease the chance of young children hiding beneath. Both the interview room at the patient site and the clinician's room at the teleprovider site should be maintained as confidential and quiet space. The space that teleproviders use will likely be construed as their offices. Thus, it will be expected to appear professional and reassure the patient that the space is confidential and family friendly. Consideration should be given to a room that is large enough to accommodate trainees.

At the patient sites, practical considerations may include placing a "Clinical Session in Progress—Quiet Please" sign on the door and informing staff about the importance of maintaining a trusted clinical space. The physical layout of the room should be considered, including limiting the possibility that the encounter could be observed through a window or that eavesdropping could occur. This consideration is sometimes challenging at sites that use the telemedicine room for multiple purposes, such as the school nurse's office. The room setup should take into consideration the target population. For example, if working with many patients presenting with ADHD, extra attention may be given limiting access to equipment or other room supplies when a child has difficulty sitting still and/or keeping their hands to themselves. If working with a potentially aggressive population, extra attention should be given to limit equipment or room components (eg, blinds) that could be torn from the walls, as well as close support from the telepresenter.

Technological Factors Affecting the Clinical Encounter

A high-quality video signal is crucial to the success of the telemental health session, with recommendations generally advising a bandwidth of greater than 384 kB per second.[4,33] High-quality audio signal also assists with identifying nuances of each other's verbal communication. The room should ideally be away from clinic and street noise because the microphones are very sensitive, and extraneous sounds can interfere with the session. Toys can produce uncomfortable levels of noise and foam blocks, books, markers, and papers may be an alternative, depending on the patient population and developmental stage.

Video quality and camera placement are also important to the quality of the telemental health session in order to clearly observe facial expressions, affect, relatedness, crying, and other nonverbal reactions. Considerations include the following[3,4]:

- To minimize shadows, lighting should emanate from behind the camera;
- Rooms with no windows or adequate window cover in order to control lighting;
- Professional colors/backgrounds consistent with typical office settings; and
- Avoidance of clothing with high contrast, such as stripes and busy patterns.

The Patient-Provider Relationship and Videoconferencing Etiquette

It is important to translate the same patient engagement and rapport building strategies to the telemental health session.[49] Shadowing existing teleproviders and consulting with colleagues often foster the teleprovider comfort level associated with strong therapeutic relationship building. Strategies used in onsite visits translate to the telemental health environment, such as noting a child wearing a shirt from a favorite team or taking time to talk about local/school events. Some teleproviders may use more animated gestures or attend more closely to nonverbal cues such as facial expressions, although overly exaggerated/fast movements/hand gestures should be kept to a minimum to avoid pixilation. Verbal communications may be more deliberate to adjust for the slight auditory lag and to clearly indicate when the teleprovider has finished speaking in order to facilitate reciprocity in communication, although this is decreasing as a less frequent concern due increasing availability of high-speed connectivity.

Families often quickly accommodate to the technology setting because of previous experience in using videoconferencing for social purposes, such as Skyping/Face Timing with friends or family members.[4] Reminders of the clinical nature of the interaction and the additional security of the videoconferencing systems are encouraged. The technology itself may be used to build rapport, such as a virtual "high 5" or holding a drawing to the camera.

Assessment

As in onsite assessment, telemental health assessment may include time with the child and adult together and individually, depending on the child's age, impulse control, verbal skills, and ability to separate from caregivers. The teleprovider often directs the telepresenter in assisting with managing who is in the room, and directing those outside the room to the waiting area or engaging children as they wait their turn. In evaluating preschoolers, it is helpful to observe the child in developmentally appropriate interactions with the support of the family, telepresenter, and other supporters such as teachers. The child may be observed in both free play and interactions with family and staff in order to assess social, motor, and verbal skills. This observation may assist in assessing the young child's level of attunement, pleasure in the interaction, or spontaneity in play. Another consideration is the child's level of cognitive development and ability to understand videoconferencing. Preschool-aged children may have difficulty with the concept that the teleprovider is a "real" person existing in a different location.[4]

Several innovative strategies are being developed to assess developmental disorders over videoconferencing. Reese's team[50] report on the utility and validity of an autism spectrum disorder assessment protocol conducted via videoconferencing. They have also developed an innovative, cost-effective Integrated Systems Using Telemedicine model for autism. This telemedicine model links students and families, trained local early intervention providers and educators at the child's school, and a team of professionals at the academic health center in order to complete comprehensive autism evaluations,[51] helping keep the child close to home.

Pharmacotherapy

Pharmacotherapy can be accomplished with consideration of clinical, regulatory, and logistical issues,[4,52] consistent with all American Academy of Child and Adolescent Psychiatry practice parameters. Approaches used in prescribing medications depend on the model being used. In one model, medication is prescribed directly by the tele-provider, most often a child psychiatrist. In another, the teleprovider manages the patient until he or she is stabilized, and care is then transferred back to the referring clinician. Finally, the telepsychiatrist may see the patient for a one-time consultation with recommendations for the referring clinician. With all models, maintaining communication with the PCP is essential. The teleprovider often requires a recent physical examination and may order additional diagnostic tests depending on the child. In order to provide medication treatment, it is necessary to perform a diagnostic evaluation before prescribing medication.

When a patient is seen for the first time, the teleprovider obtains consent that acknowledges that the family has the right to seek out in-person treatment should they choose.[31] Teleproviders should review the procedures for medication prescribing and obtaining refills. Prescriptions that are not controlled can be ordered by calling the pharmacy, written and mailed, or e-prescribed. E-prescribing, which fits logistically with telemental health, is an increasing practice. Controlled substances such as schedule II stimulants have more regulatory constraints and cannot be refilled or called to the pharmacy. Stimulant prescriptions can be mailed directly to patients' homes or their pharmacies. Some sites may require that prescriptions be mailed to the patient site for distribution to families, or that copies of prescriptions be maintained according to the specifications of a Medicaid contract or other regulations. E-prescribing of stimulants is also an option in some venues because the Drug Enforcement Administration (DEA) approved the electronic prescription of controlled substances. This DEA-sanctioned practice is approved in most states, but adoption has been slower than e-prescribing in general, likely because of the security restrictions and collaboration requirements (Department of Justice, DEA, Office of Diversion Control: http://www.deadiversion.usdoj.gov/ecomm/e_rx/). In addition, teleproviders should monitor federal updates related to prescribing controlled medications and the Ryan Haight Online Pharmacy Consumer Protection Act of 2008.

Medication monitoring is also possible via telepsychiatry and should be followed according to the same standards of care as in-person psychiatric management.[52] Staff at the patient site can obtain vital signs, height, and weight on the patient as well as the Abnormal Involuntary Movement Scale. Laboratory tests and electrocardiograms may also be obtained. For care between telemental health sessions, teleproviders assist with clear direction and contact numbers for interim needs such as requesting refills, asking questions, and reporting adverse effects. Protocols describing this process help to ensure safe monitoring of medications and to define expectations for staff at both sites. Families should be educated about this policy and given adequate time for refill requests to prevent running out of medications.

SUMMARY

Telemental health services with youth will likely continue to grow because of the increasing workforce gaps between need and service across behavioral health specialties as well as the call for new models of family-centered care and collaboration across child-serving systems. Ideally, they also assist with 2-generation needs such as onsite and telemedicine services that also address parent/family health needs. National and state initiatives continue to work to address regulatory/legal barriers to telemedicine in general, including efforts around interstate licensure and parity. Although technology advances and improved connectivity open many doors to expand telemental health, the defining *why*, *what*, *when*, *who*, *where*, and *how* will remain key considerations in delivering effective interventions.

Going forward, expanded telemental health services to children and adolescents will be supported by the continued evolution of secure, high-speed, mobile videoconferencing options across the range of current and future devices. Technology advances will further expand telemental health service delivery sites, including unsupervised settings such as the home and youth mobile devices. With this expansion comes the need for careful consideration and evaluation of services to maximize benefit for youth and families, minimize risk, and optimally support community stakeholders to test models of care, to evaluate quality improvement efforts, and to examine the effectiveness of services delivered through telemental health across diverse populations.

With an at times overwhelming array of technology options to assess and treat child behavioral health concerns (synchronous mental health/videoconferencing, social media, asynchronous mental health, mHealth, virtual technologies, virtual reality, augmented reality, intelligent wearable devices, and artificial intelligence), it is essential that teams of experts (eg, clinicians, health information technologists, informatics leaders, evaluators, patient advocates, and others) work together to carefully match the best technology options for the specific needs of youth and their families.[53,54] With these exciting new options comes continued need for guidance from professional organizations and for careful consideration of training to support teleproviders around competencies to provide the safest and most effective pediatric services.

ACKNOWLEDGMENTS

The authors appreciate the editorial assistance of graduate student Ms Natasia Adams.

REFERENCES

1. Perou R, Bitsko RH, Blumberg SJ, et al. Mental health surveillance among children—United States, 2005-2011. MMWR Suppl 2013;62(2):1–35.
2. Merikangas KR, He JP, Burstein M, et al. Service utilization for lifetime mental disorders in U.S. adolescents: results of the National Comorbidity Survey-Adolescent Supplement (NCS-A). J Am Acad Child Adolesc Psychiatry 2011; 50(1):32–45.
3. Luxton D, Nelson E, Maheu M. A practitioner's guide to telemental health: how to conduct legal, ethical, and evidence-based telepractice. Washington, DC: American Psychological Association Press; 2016.
4. Cain S, Nelson E, Myers K. Telemental health. In: Dulcan MK, editor. Dulcan's textbook of child and adolescent psychiatry. Washington, DC: American Psychiatric Publishing; 2015. p. 1–18.
5. Myers K, Turvey C, editors. Telemental health: clinical, technical and administrative foundation for evidence-based practice. London: Elsevier; 2012.
6. Comer JS, Barlow DH. The occasional case against broad dissemination and implementation: retaining a role for specialty care in the delivery of psychological treatments. Am Psychol 2014;69(1):1–18.

7. Smalley B, Warren J, Rainer J, editors. Rural mental health: issues, policies, and best practices. New York: Springer; 2012.
8. Gloff NE, Lenoue SR, Novins DK, et al. Telemental health for children and adolescents. Int Rev Psychiatry 2015;27(6):513–24.
9. Nelson EL, Bui T. Rural telepsychology services for children and adolescents. J Clin Psychol 2010;66(5):490–501.
10. Arora S, Thornton K, Komaromy M, et al. Demonopolizing medical knowledge. Acad Med 2014;89(1):30–2.
11. Myers KM, Valentine JM, Melzer SM. Feasibility, acceptability, and sustainability of telepsychiatry for children and adolescents. Psychiatr Serv 2007;58(11): 1493–6.
12. Yellowlees PM, Hilty DM, Marks SL, et al. A retrospective analysis of a child and adolescent eMental Health program. J Am Acad Child Adolesc Psychiatry 2008; 47(1):103–7.
13. Myers KM, Sulzbacher S, Melzer SM. Telepsychiatry with children and adolescents: are patients comparable to those evaluated in usual outpatient care? Telemed J E Health 2004;10(3):278–85.
14. Hilty DM, Ferrer DC, Parish MB, et al. The effectiveness of telemental health: a 2013 review. Telemed J E Health 2013;19(6):444–54.
15. Bashshur RL, Shannon GW, Bashshur N, et al. The empirical evidence for telemedicine interventions in mental disorders. Telemed J E Health 2016;22(2):87–113.
16. Nelson E, Sharp S. Telemental health update. Pediatr Clin North Am 2016;63(5): 913–31.
17. Marcin JP, Nesbitt TS, Cole SL, et al. Changes in diagnosis, treatment, and clinical improvement among patients receiving telemedicine consultations. Telemed J E Health 2005;11(1):36–43.
18. Boydell KM, Volpe T, Kertes A, et al. A review of the outcomes of the recommendations made during paediatric telepsychiatry consultations. J Telemed Telecare 2007;13(6):277–81.
19. Myers K, Vander Stoep A, Zhou C, et al. Effectiveness of a telehealth service delivery model for treating attention-deficit/hyperactivity disorder: a community-based randomized controlled trial. J Am Acad Child Adolesc Psychiatry 2015; 54(4):263–74.
20. Vander Stoep A, McCarty CA, Zhou C, et al. The children's attention-deficit hyperactivity disorder telemental health treatment study: caregiver outcomes. J Abnorm Child Psychol 2016. [Epub ahead of print].
21. Nelson EL, Patton S. Using videoconferencing to deliver individual therapy and pediatric psychology interventions with children and adolescents. J Child Adolesc Psychopharmacol 2016;26(3):212–20.
22. Duncan AB, Velasquez SE, Nelson EL. Using videoconferencing to provide psychological services to rural children and adolescents: a review and case example. J Clin Child Adolesc Psychol 2014;43(1):115–27.
23. Gros DF, Morland LA, Greene CJ, et al. Delivery of evidence-based psychotherapy via video telehealth. J Psychopathol Behav Assess 2013;35(4):506–21.
24. Nelson E, Duncan A. Cognitive-behavioral therapy using televideo. Cogn Behav Pract 2015;22(3):269–80.
25. Davis AM, Sampilo M, Gallagher KC, et al. Treating rural pediatric obesity through telemedicine vs. telephone: outcomes from a cluster randomized controlled trial. J Telemed Telecare 2016;22(2):86–95.
26. Lambert D, Gale J, Hartley D, et al. Understanding the business case for telemental health in rural communities. J Behav Health Serv Res 2016;43:366–79.

27. Shore JH, Manson SM. A developmental model for rural telepsychiatry. Psychiatr Serv 2005;56(8):976–80.

28. American Telemedicine Association. State telemedicine gaps analysis: coverage & reimbursement. 2015. Available at: http://www.americantelemed.org/docs/default-source/policy/50-state-telemedicine-gaps-analysis--coverage-and-reimbursement.pdf. Accessed June 12, 2016.

29. American Telemedicine Association. State telemedicine gaps analysis: coverage & reimbursement–parity laws for private insurance. 2015. Available at: http://www.americantelemed.org/docs/default-source/policy/ata-map-telemedicine-parity-2014-3-7.pdf. Accessed June 12, 2016.

30. Hilty DM, Schoemaker EZ, Myers K, et al. Need for and steps toward a clinical guideline for the telemental health care of children and adolescents. J Child Adolesc Psychopharmacol 2016;26(3):283–95.

31. American Academy of Child and Adolescent Psychiatry. Committee on quality issues. Practice parameter for child and adolescent telepsychiatry. 2008. Available at: www.jaacap.com/content/pracparam. Accessed June 12, 2016.

32. American Psychological Association. Guidelines for the practice of telepsychology. 2013. Available at: http://www.apa.org/practice/guidelines/telepsychology.aspx. Accessed June 12, 2016.

33. Grady BJ, Myers KM, Nelson EL, et al. Evidence-based practice for telemental health. Telemed J E Health 2011;17(2):131–48.

34. Turvey C, Coleman M, Dennison O, et al. ATA practice guidelines for video-based online mental health services. Telemed J E Health 2013;19(9):722–30.

35. Kramer GM, Luxton DD. Telemental health for children and adolescents: an overview of legal, regulatory, and risk management issues. J Child Adolesc Psychopharmacol 2016;26(3):198–203.

36. Myers K, Comer JS. The case for telemental health for improving the accessibility and quality of children's mental health services. J Child Adolesc Psychopharmacol 2016;26(3):186–91.

37. Goldstein F, Myers K. Telemental health: a new collaboration for pediatricians and child psychiatrists. Pediatr Ann 2014;43(2):79–84.

38. McWilliams JK. Integrating telemental healthcare with the patient-centered medical home model. J Child Adolesc Psychopharmacol 2016;26(3):278–82.

39. Stephan S, Lever N, Bernstein L, et al. Telemental health in schools. J Child Adolesc Psychopharmacol 2016;26(3):266–72.

40. Nelson EL, Duncan AB, Peacock G, et al. Telemedicine and adherence to national guidelines for ADHD evaluation: a case study. Psychol Serv 2012;9(3):293–7.

41. Bastastini A. Improving rehabilitative efforts for juvenile offenders through the use of telemental healthcare. J Child Adolesc Psychopharmacol 2016;26(3):273–7.

42. Crum KI, Comer JS. Using synchronous videoconferencing to deliver family-based mental healthcare. J Child Adolesc Psychopharmacol 2016;26(3):229–34.

43. Nelson EL, Fennel S, Sosland J, et al. Telepsychology best practices in translating evidence-based services for child trauma to the home. Poster presented at: the National Conference in Clinical Child & Adolescent Psychology: translating research into practice. Lawrence, KS, October 1, 2014.

44. Smith C, Piamjariyakul U, Werkowitch M, et al. A clinical trial of translation of evidence based interventions to mobile tablets and illness specific internet sites. Int J Sens Netw Data Commun 2016;5(1) [pii:138].

45. Hilty DM, Crawford A, Teshima J, et al. A framework for telepsychiatric training and e-health: competency-based education, evaluation and implications. Int Rev Psychiatry 2015;27(6):569–92.
46. Szeftel R, Mandelbaum S, Sullman-Smith H, et al. Telepsychiatry for children with developmental disabilities: applications for patient care and medical education. Child Adolesc Psychiatr Clin N Am 2011;20(1):95–111.
47. Nelson EL, Bui T, Sharp S. Telemental health competencies: training examples from a youth depression telemedicine clinic. In: Gregerson M, editor. Technology innovations for behavioral education. New York: Springer; 2011. p. 41–8.
48. American Telemedicine Association. Expert consensus recommendation: videoconferencing-based telepresenting. 2011. Available at: http://www.american telemed.org/docs/default-source/standards/expert-consensus-recommendations-for-videoconferencing-based-telepresenting.pdf. Accessed June 12, 2016.
49. Goldstein F, Glueck D. Developing rapport and therapeutic alliance during tele-mental health sessions with children and adolescents. J Child Adolesc Psycho-pharmacol 2016;26(3):204–11.
50. Reese RM, Jamison TR, Braun M, et al. Brief report: use of interactive television in identifying autism in young children: methodology and preliminary data. J Autism Dev Disord 2015;45(5):1474–82.
51. Reese RM, Braun MJ, Hoffmeier S, et al. Preliminary evidence for the integrated systems using telemedicine. Telemed J E Health 2015;21(7):581–7.
52. Cain S, Sharp S. Telepharmacotherapy for children and adolescent psychiatric patients. J Child Adolesc Psychopharmacol 2016;26(3):221–8.
53. Mohr DC, Burns MN, Schueller SM, et al. Behavioral intervention technologies: evidence review and recommendations for future research in mental health. Gen Hosp Psychiatry 2013;35(4):332–8.
54. Hilty DM, Yellowlees PM. Collaborative mental health services using multiple technologies: the new way to practice and a new standard of practice? J Am Acad Child Adolesc Psychiatry 2015;54(4):245–6.

Teaching Child and Adolescent Psychiatry in the Twenty-First Century

A Reflection on the Role of Technology in Education

Shih Yee-Marie Tan Gipson, MD[a,b],*, Jung Won Kim, MD[a,b],
Ah Lahm Shin, MD[c], Robert Kitts, MD[a], Eleni Maneta, MD[a,b],[1]

KEYWORDS

- Child and adolescent psychiatry fellowship • Technology • Media • Education
- Millennial learner

KEY POINTS

- Technology is infiltrating graduate medical education, including child and adolescent psychiatry (CAP) fellowship training.
- Technology can be used to enhance teaching and improve administrative tasks.
- Learning about technology through an informatics curriculum is also an important part of CAP fellowship training.
- Although there are many advantages to using technology in education, there are also some challenges that should be considered.
- Further research is needed to better understand the impacts of technology on CAP training.

INTRODUCTION

As part of the digital revolution, there has been a large change in the technology landscape in all industries and sectors, including medicine. The mobility and accessibility of technology has also made an impact on education, which is now targeted toward

Conflict of Interest: The authors have no conflict of interest to disclose.
 a Department of Psychiatry, Harvard Medical School, 25, Shattuck Street, Boston, MA 02115, USA; b Department of Psychiatry, Boston Children's Hospital, 300 Longwood Avenue, Boston, MA 02115, USA; c Department of Anesthesia, Boston Children's Hospital, 300 Longwood Avenue, Boston, MA 02115, USA
[1] Senior Author.
* Corresponding author.
E-mail address: Marie.Gipson@childrens.harvard.edu

the new generation of learners, born between 1981 and 2004, and commonly referred to as millennial learners.

Millennial learners have a deep understanding and preference for technology[1,2] and process information differently than previous generations of learners.[3] Although general medical education and general residencies, including psychiatric residencies, are well underway toward a millennial curriculum,[3,4] less attention has been paid to subspecialty training, including child and adolescent psychiatry (CAP) fellowships.

The purpose of this article is to review the use of technology in teaching CAP fellows in the twenty-first century and to examine the advantages and disadvantages of incorporating such technology in fellowship training. Three areas of focus is discussed in terms of how technology can impact CAP fellowship training: the use of technology to enhance teaching and learning, the use of technology to enhance fellowship administration, and finally the importance of a technology curriculum that focuses on teaching the next generation of CAP clinician educators about educational and clinical uses of technology. Literature from general medical and psychiatric education as well as literature on the basic principles of learning is reviewed in order to help move CAP fellowship training forward.

Please note that any of the media and technologies mentioned in the article do not reflect an endorsement by the authors but are used because they are more commonly known examples to illustrate a teaching point.

TECHNOLOGY AND TEACHING

One of the most important reasons to incorporate technology in CAP training is to enhance the learning process of fellows, who are asked to take in significant amounts of new information in the span of 2 clinically challenging and busy years. Teaching CAP fellows follows the principles of adult learning theory, which postulates that adults learn best through experiential techniques; they require goal-directed and relevancy-oriented information and learn best when multiple teaching formats are combined.[5,6] Technology provides many opportunities to apply these basic adult-learning principles to CAP education. Not only can it facilitate instruction[7] but it can also help bring the teacher and the learner closer through collaborative learning and active engagement.[8] Hilty[7] describes how technology can fall within an educational triangle that is formed between teacher, learner, and subject in order to enhance both the learning and teaching processes. In this section, the authors review examples of technologies that have been used to aid adult learning; they do not focus on technologies that can only be used in the process of passive learning through lecturing, such as slide-based presentations.

One of the earliest technologies to be used in undergraduate and graduate medical education was cinematography. Blasco and colleagues[9] discuss how the use of films in a curriculum can not only improve reflections and learning across students but can also improve the educator's teaching skills. The investigators argue that using films to teach can link learning to experiences and, therefore, promote reflective learning among students.[9]

Films and now television can be useful in teaching about various aspects of human development and mental health. Akram and colleagues[10] found that using films to teach psychiatry can demonstrate a lively picture while illustrating the course of an illness, thus, allowing students the opportunity to observe mock cases to help deepen their understanding of various psychiatric disorders. Hankir and colleagues[11] also examined the use of films in teachings about mental health and conclude that using film can aid in the dissolution of stigma associated with psychiatric disorders, such as schizophrenia. They also described how teaching through films presents a great advantage as it can illustrate a clinical picture that can traverse through time and place, without the need to consider issues such as confidentiality.[11]

An example of how films can be used to assist with teaching in child psychiatry is the *Normal Development Video Series: A Longitudinal Stimulation Video Curriculum Resource for Educators* developed by child and adolescent psychiatrist Geri Fox MD. This film series provides a selection of key moments from 2 children's development over 20 years and can be used to teach normal development. The *Up Series* is a more mainstream series of documentary films that have been following the lives of 14 British children since 1964, when they were 7 years old. There are currently 8 films (one every 7 years), with the most recent being *56 UP*. Finally, *Thin* is another documentary that revolves around 4 women with eating disorders, including one 15 year old being treated at one of the Renfrew Center eating disorder treatment facilities. These examples are a few of the plethora of media relevant to child psychiatry that could be used for teaching.

The use of films in teaching about clinical scenarios has now been taken one step further with the introduction of virtual patients as teachers. Web-based simulations including virtual patients are already being used for training in various aspects of the health care field. One of the main advantages of Web-based simulations is that they provide the opportunity to practice clinical skills and problem solving in settings that simulate real patient encounters but that may represent less anxiety-provoking situations.[12] Although, compared with other specialties, psychiatry was challenging in terms of simulating affective and behavioral processes needed to mimic disorders,[13] more recently studies have demonstrated encouraging results in terms of the use of virtual patients for training in the mental health field.[14,15] For example, Gorrindo and colleagues[13] successfully developed and used a computer simulation assessment tool to teach psychiatric residents how to obtain consent for treatment with antipsychotics. The tool was designed using custom Web-based simulation software, Flash-based video, and a standard Web browser. To the authors' knowledge virtual patients have not been studied in CAP fellowship training; their use, however, would offer fellows the opportunity to practice their clinical skills across the developmental spectrum and receive feedback in a more structured way. It would also ensure that fellows get access to children of all ages and with all possible conditions, which, depending on the site of training, may not be feasible to achieve with live patients.

Web-based learning, or e-learning, is also infiltrating psychiatric education and should be considered in CAP fellowship training. E-learning represents a learner-centered approach, whereby the learner is in control of how and when he or she reviews the material.[16] E-learning is usually incorporated into the curriculum; however, the context in which it is used will determine its effectiveness.[17] Curricula that incorporate e-learning can vary in terms of how much they rely on online activities compared with face-to-face activities with peers and teachers; this also depends on the goals of the course and whether the focus is more on accessing material or participating in joint activities around learning.[16] A less directed form of e-learning also exists, which involves self-driven utilization of the Web to research various topics. Evidence is already accumulating that a significant portion of residents in varying fields, including psychiatry, are relying more heavily on online sources, such as PubMed or UpToDate, than on textbooks or other printed material.[18] Although the equivalent learning patterns have not been studied in CAP fellows, it can be assumed that they would be similar. The usage of online or e-materials highlights the importance of carefully implementing e-learning methods into CAP fellowship training. Similar to research literacy, CAP fellows would benefit from more formalized education on how to assess the quality of online resources pertaining to CAP and also how to engage patients and families around it given the abundance of both misinformation and helpful information.

One of the most important aspects of adult learning includes active participation, and advances in technology have significantly enhanced the way in which that can be pursued. Audience response systems (ARS) or personal response systems (eg, Poll Everywhere, Socrative, and Mentimeter) are devices specifically designed to elicit active, and usually anonymous, participation from the audience during a session. Certain applications (apps) will also provide the capability of questioning knowledge taught outside of the teaching session in a gamelike competitive fashion among learners to promote further active participation. Boscardin and Penuel[19] reviewed the literature on the use of ARS in learning and found evidence to support the notion that ARS enhance audience participation and can also play a role in formative assessment of the instruction. Interestingly, however, they did not find clear evidence to suggest that ARS use enhances knowledge acquisition, although there is indirect evidence linking active participation and knowledge gains. A more recent study by Hettinger and colleagues[20] looked at the implementation of ARS in psychiatric training and particularly in preparation for the Psychiatry Residency In-Training Examination (PRITE). The investigators concluded that the addition of ARS to the PRITE preparation resulted in a significant improvement in test scores, therefore, highlighting the utility of the system in a concrete fashion. Given these results, ARS show promise for use in CAP fellowship training as well, particularly because CAP fellows are expected to digest large amounts of new information in the relatively short period of time that spans the fellowship.

An aspect of teaching unique to psychiatry is the teaching that comes in the form of psychotherapy supervision. Although the role of technology in psychotherapy supervision is less clear, Watkins[21] argues that it has the potential to enhance the value of the supervisee's experience. The investigator reviews possible ways in which technology can aid in supervision, from digital recordings of sessions and live webcams to the use of virtual reality patients to practice skills before entering the psychotherapeutic relationship. He concludes that psychotherapy supervision in the new millennium will most definitely take advantage of technological advances.[21] Similarly one would expect the same to be true for subspecialties of psychiatry, including CAP. Chlebowski and Fremont[22] have already argued for the value of webcams both in supervision of CAP fellows and also for case presentations. Additionally, if these recordings are used in teaching of medical students, they can assist in recruitment efforts by providing an opportunity for medical students to get a better sense of what many child psychiatrists do, because the nature of the psychotherapeutic relationship may preclude students from being able to sit in on an alluring therapeutic session.

Finally, technology can enhance teaching by promoting access to and sharing of educational material, thereby, assisting busy CAP educators with limited local resources. The Association of American Medical Colleges' (AAMC) MedEdPORTAL[23] is a free, open-access publication service on health education teachings and assessment resources and provides peer-reviewed curricula. Another example that is specific to CAP is the International Association for Child and Adolescent Psychiatry and Allied Professions' (IACAPAP) online *Textbook of Child and Adolescent Mental Health*,[24] which is free and accessible to anyone throughout the world. It includes articles, video links, and even PowerPoint presentations for teaching. It even includes 2 articles related to technology, "Problematic Internet Use" and "e-Therapy: Using Computer and Mobile Technologies in Treatment." The American Academy of Child and Adolescent Psychiatry's (AACAP) Web site is also host to the "Child and Adolescent Psychiatry Resources for Medical Student Educators,"[25] which is a toolbox of online resources for educators to use, including multiple PowerPoint lectures by child psychiatrists throughout the United States. Additionally, online educational video modules can assist with teaching and even be used for assignments in a flipped classroom approach, such as the following Web sites: National Neuroscience Curriculum Initiative (http://www.nncionline.org/) and Cold Spring Harbor Laboratory's Genes to Cognition Online (http://www.g2conline.org/).

TECHNOLOGY AND ADMINISTRATION

A less recognized role of technology in CAP fellowship training is its role in administrative tasks, such as scheduling, organization, evaluations, and so forth. Although these aspects of training are not directly related to learning, they can definitely facilitate the process. Ellaway and Masters[16] discuss the importance of technology in supporting the learning environment particularly in medicine. For example, the investigators note that technology can assist with scheduling rotations, tracking content and participants, enhancing communication and file sharing, and most importantly assisting in auditing, quality assurance, and compliance with regulations set forth by governing bodies, such as the AAMC.[16]

An administrative task most closely related to training is that of ensuring timely bidirectional evaluation and feedback to and from trainees. Historically evaluations had been collected on paper, which required considerable administrative effort and posed challenges in terms of ensuring compliance by all parties, dealing with missing or lost papers, and then compiling the feedback into performance reports and tracking trainees' progress.[26] Electronic forms of assessment, on the other hand, can provide more information, using built-in algorithms and programming that can compile raw data and allow for easy monitoring of compliance.

In 2006, Benjamin and colleagues[27] reviewed Web-based systems for assessment and evaluation of trainees and found that, compared with paper methods, online assessment tools not only provide information on trainees' competence but also provide feedback on the quality of teaching and the learning environment. Similarly, online evaluation systems for faculty teaching have also shown advantages over traditional paper forms. Natt and colleagues[26] found that residents were significantly more likely to return faculty evaluations (return rate increased from 35% to 90%) when using an online evaluation system. One of the most important reasons behind this increase was the ease of the completion and submission process. At the same time, the higher response rates by residents resulted in more faculty making changes to their teaching style based on feedback they received.

Reynolds and colleagues[28] took the electronic feedback process one step further by implementing a portable electronic system using a Quick Response code reader (QR reader) that generated a brief evaluation for obstetrics and gynecology residents. The evaluation was conducted immediately postoperatively, reviewed with the resident, and transmitted to the training office. The investigators reported that use of this tool resulted in a 64% increase in evaluation completions and noted that it represents an effective tool to provide immediate formative feedback to trainees.

More recently, Havel and colleagues[29] implemented a 5-item mobile survey conducted on smartphones to help psychiatry residents evaluate their classes and to capture attendance. Similar to prior studies, they noted a 10-fold increase in the number of completed evaluation; but more importantly, they also noted an increase in class participation from 64% in 2014 to 81% in 2015, presumably due to improvements in the classes after resident feedback.

Regular evaluations and feedback are of paramount importance in any training program, and child psychiatry is no exception to that. As described earlier, an electronic-based evaluation system can increase participation and rates of return and lead to important changes within the program, all with an interface that most trainees and faculty are generally satisfied with. Further, it can also assist program directors in providing useful longitudinal feedback that captures progress, both to their trainees and to their faculty, while at the same time fulfilling important administrative requirements set forth by the Accreditation Council for Graduate Medical Education (ACGME).

Technology can also facilitate scheduling and duty-hour monitoring tasks within training programs, including CAP fellowships. Programs, such as Am I On (http://www.amion.com/) or New Innovations (https://www.new-innov.com/pub/), can be used to schedule rotations and call coverage and also monitor how many hours trainees are working to help prevent fatigue and duty-hour violations, both of which can have a negative impact on training and education.

Ultimately technology in any training program, including CAP fellowship, can help streamline administrative tasks and ensure their completion in a timely fashion with the least amount of effort necessary, thereby with the least amount of disruption to training otherwise.

CREATING A TECHNOLOGY CURRICULUM

Apart from using technology to facilitate learning and administrative tasks, a CAP fellowship is also responsible for teaching the new generation of child psychiatrists how to appropriately use technology in patient care and education. Huang and Alessi[30] have been arguing about the need for an informatics curriculum for psychiatry since 1998. These investigators review 4 major areas of focus that would be covered in such a curriculum: use of technology in direct patient care, in communication with patients and other clinicians, in education about psychiatry, and in the management of a clinical practice. A technology curriculum in CAP fellowship should not be expected to cover all innovations available at a given time; rather, it should consider focusing on providing the following:

- An understanding of the general landscape of technology that is currently available in child psychiatry
- Consumer literacy on how to approach a new technology (eg, Mobile apps, wearable technology, and so forth) advertised as being beneficial to patients or practice, such as cost, benefit, alternatives, and evidence
- Research literacy on the impact that technology may have on development and mental health
- An understanding of how these tools can fit into daily practice for the purposes of diagnosis, monitoring of symptoms, treatment, patient communication, and continuing education

One of the most discussed technological advances in patient care, and one that should be incorporated into a CAP informatics curriculum, is telepsychiatry. Despite existing evidence that supports its use in clinical practice,[31] telepsychiatry has not been fully incorporated into curricula. Sunderji and colleagues[32] highlight the need for an evidence-based approach to telepsychiatry training and point to the lack of clear guidelines and competencies that address learning needs. Training CAP fellows in telepsychiatry increases the likelihood that they would incorporate it into their practice, which can have important implications in terms of improving disparities in access to care both due to geographic reasons but also due to language barriers and cultural reasons.[32,33]

As part of a technology curriculum, CAP fellows should also be familiar with the literature on the intersection of technology, development, and mental health. Patients, families, primary care providers, and schools may have a broad range of questions from how to promote cyber safety to identifying problematic Internet use to when to introduce technology to their children. The Boston Children's Hospital's Center on Media and Child Health[34] has a free digital library that contains more than 3500 article citations about the effects of media on children and adolescents.

A technology curriculum will not be complete without including ethical and professional considerations that involve the use of technology in patient care. This becomes particularly important in child psychiatry whereby appropriate boundaries may be less clear to begin with[35,36] and whereby the patients are significantly more likely to be using technology as a means of communication (social media, blogging, and so forth). When thinking about professionalism in relation to technology in CAP practice, there are 2 broad categories that should be considered. The first category involves issues that are directly related to patient care, such as patient privacy, boundary violations, and so forth. DeJong and colleagues[37] identify the following important topics that should be addressed with trainees: liability around new technologies that are used to interface with patients (eg, e-mail), confidentiality with regards to social-media posts that may advertently or inadvertently give away protected information about patients, safety issues that may come up by researching patients online, and netiquette in terms of electronic communication. The second category involves issues that pertain to the online identity of the physician and how that may indirectly affect patient care. Online content about the physician may be brought into psychotherapy, thus, affecting neutrality or, if negative, it may even undermine the physician's professional identity.[37,38] Both categories have to be covered during CAP training; professionalism issues regarding technology should be made explicit, particularly because there may be transgenerational differences in recognizing them.

Another aspect that should be considered when teaching CAP fellows about technology is how to approach its use within the patient-doctor relationship. From the moment the clinician meets patients, technology may play a role in alliance and understanding patients. How would an initial interview be different if a clinician entered the room and asked the teen to immediately put his or her cell phone away as opposed to waiting a little while and asking what he or she was doing on the phone in an inquisitive and respectful manner? Or what if the clinician had his or her eyes on the computer most of the session? While collecting the social history, there is the opportunity to ask about technology use (amount of time spent, level of surveillance, and so forth). Is technology a potential port of entry into getting to know patients more? What does patients' social platform say about their self-identify and self-expression? By inquiring about the use of technology, would this increase the likelihood of patients bringing up related stressors, such as cyber bullying? Would a middle school child engage more with therapy that involved technology, such as a video game to assist with learning how to relax? It is hoped that raising such questions will prompt CAP fellows to be more thoughtful of the role technology.

Finally, CAP fellows should be educated, whether it is through their actual clinical rotations or a transition to practice, on how to choose an approach technology within a larger system of care and as if they were establishing an independent practice. Given the rapidly growing and evolving field of health information technology, AACAP's Task Force on Health Information and Technology was developed to assist AACAP members in understanding the field and its application in the practice of CAP and to promote informed use for the purpose of improving the clinical service and quality for patients. AACAP's Web site provides information on electronic medical records and how to choose one along with this task force's policy statement, "Confidentiality in Health Information and Technology."[39]

In summary, a technology curriculum could be developed along the framework of the ACGME's core competencies with regard to technology and its growing relationship to patient care, medical knowledge, practice-based learning and improvement, interpersonal and communication skills, professionalism, and systems-based practice in CAP.

CHALLENGES AND PITFALLS

Although technology can be an invaluable tool for CAP training, it is important to recognize that it also presents with challenges that may limit its applicability. First and foremost is the question about access to technology. E-learning presumes access to the proper devices, such as laptops, tablets, and smartphones. It also requires access to the Internet, which, through a mobile device, involves data usage–related charges. Overreliance on technology can, therefore, potentially create unequal learning opportunities, leaving those with less means behind. Until universal access is addressed, alternate methods of teaching should remain available, so that all trainees can have an equal opportunity in education. Another pitfall of overly relying on technology for training purposes is that it can malfunction. Internet dead zones, technical problems with devices, data loss, and so forth can interfere with learning and demotivate trainees.

Another challenge with the use of technology in CAP training is the direct and indirect effects that it can have on learning. More and more research has been documenting the negative effects of technology use on attention, particularly when it comes to learning.[40,41] Using mobile devices or laptops with access to social media apps, instant messaging, or text messaging capabilities during a teaching session has the potential to distract from the learning process. In addition, there are also some data to support that technology may impact how our brains process information. A study by Mueller and Oppenheimer[42] determined that taking notes on a laptop leads to shallower processing of information and worse performance in conceptual questions compared with taking notes by hand. The investigators attributed this difference to the fact that the ease and speed of using a laptop to take notes leads to mindless transcribing of content rather than synthesizing and summarizing. Technology also affects learning by engaging multiple senses simultaneously; although multisensory learning is considered superior,[43] there is also evidence to suggest that it can eventually lead to an overload of information and worse performance.[44]

Separate from the considerations on learning, technology can also have adverse effects on mental and physical health, which too have to be taken into account before encouraging increased use during CAP training. Two new terms have been coined to describe the effects of technology overuse on mental health, *telepressure* and *fear of missing out*, which refer to the urge to respond to notifications on electronic devices and are associated with higher levels of burnout, stress, and poor sleep hygiene.[45] At the same time there are also multiple studies describing the negative impact of continuous exposure to technology on physical health.[46,47]

SUMMARY

Technology is already becoming an integral part of graduate medical education, and CAP fellowship training will be no exception to that. As described earlier, there are numerous advantages to incorporating technological advances to CAP training, particularly because it addresses a generation of millennial learners. A technology and informatics psychiatry curriculum also addresses the needs of the younger generation of patients who may be more receptive to using technology for their care but who may not be aware of the confidentiality and privacy pitfalls associated with its use.

There are still many unknowns as to how to best incorporate technology into CAP training. Ongoing research and discussion is necessary to shed light on how technology affects fellowship training and its relationship to patient care. However, we can maximize its advantages and minimize its disadvantages by becoming more familiar with the field, including its existing and growing body of research literature as well as how it is being approached by organizations in child psychiatry (eg, IACAPAP and AACAP) and those outside (eg, American Psychiatric Association, American Association of Directors of Psychiatric Residency, and AAMC) who may have more experience and knowledge.

REFERENCES

1. Roberts DH, Newman LR, Schwartzstein RM. Twelve tips for facilitating millennials' learning. Med Teach 2012;34(4):274–8.
2. Revell SM, McCurry MK. Engaging millennial learners: effectiveness of personal response system technology with nursing students in small and large classrooms. J Nurs Educ 2010;49(5):272–5.
3. Phitayakorn R, Nick MW, Alseidi A, et al. WISE-MD usage among millennial medical students. Am J Surg 2015;209(1):152–7.
4. Hilty D, Alverson DC, Alpert JE, et al. Virtual reality, telemedicine, web and data processing innovations in medical and psychiatric education and clinical care. Acad Psychiatry 2006;30:528–33.
5. Zisook S, Benjamin S, Balon R, et al. Alternate methods of teaching psychopharmacology. Acad Psychiatry 2005;29:141–54.
6. Knowles MS, Holton EF III, Swanson RA. The adult learner: the definitive classic in adult education and human resources development. New York: Routledge; 2014.
7. Hilty DM. Technology in psychiatric education: the technology innovation column. Acad Psychiatry 2016;40(3):543–5.
8. Black CD, Watties-Daniels AD. Cutting edge technology to enhance nursing classroom instruction at Coppin State University. ABNF J 2006;17:103–6.
9. Blasco PG, Moreto G, Blasco MG, et al. Education through movies: improving teaching skills and fostering reflection among students and teachers. Journal of Learning through the Arts 2015;11(1).
10. Akram A, O'Brien A, O'Neill A, et al. Crossing the line–learning psychiatry at the movies. Int Rev Psychiatry 2009;21(3):267–8.
11. Hankir A, Holloway D, Zaman R, et al. Cinematherapy and film as an educational tool in undergraduate psychiatry teaching: a case report and review of the literature. Psychiatr Danub 2015;27(Suppl 1):136–42.
12. Zary N, Johnson G, Boberg J, et al. Development, implementation and pilot evaluation of a web-based virtual patient case simulation environment–Web-SP. BMC Med Educ 2006;6:10.
13. Gorrindo T, Baer L, Sanders K, et al. Web-based simulation in psychiatry residency training: a pilot study. Acad Psychiatry 2011;35:232–7.
14. Sunnqvist C, Karlsson K, Lindell L, et al. Virtual patient simulation in psychiatric care - a pilot study of digital support for collaborate learning. Nurse Educ Pract 2016;17:30–5.

15. Wilkening GL, Gannon JM, Ross C, et al. Evaluation of branched-narrative virtual patients for interprofessional education of psychiatry residents. Acad Psychiatry 2016. [Epub ahead of print].
16. Ellaway R, Masters K. AMEE guide 32: e-learning in medical education part 1: learning, teaching and assessment. Med Teach 2008;30(5):455–73.
17. Ellaway RH, Pusic M, Yavner S, et al. Context matters: emergent variability in an effectiveness trial of online teaching modules. Med Educ 2014;48(4):386–96.
18. Torous J, Franzan J, O'Connor R, et al. Psychiatry residents' use of educational websites: a pilot survey study. Acad Psychiatry 2015;39(6):630–3.
19. Boscardin C, Penuel W. Exploring benefits of audience-response systems on learning: a review of the literature. Acad Psychiatry 2012;36(5):401–7.
20. Hettinger A, Spurgeon J, El-Mallakh R, et al. Using audience response system technology and PRITE questions to improve psychiatric residents' medical knowledge. Acad Psychiatry 2014;38(2):205–8.
21. Watkins CE. Psychotherapy supervision in the new millennium: competency-based, evidence-based, particularized, and energized. J Contemp Psychother 2011;42(3):193–203.
22. Chlebowski S, Fremont W. Therapeutic uses of the webcam in chid psychiatry. Acad Psychiatry 2011;35:263–7.
23. Association of American Medical Colleges. MedEdPORTAL. Available at: https://www.mededportal.org/. Accessed May 31, 2016.
24. International Association for Child and Adolescent Psychiatry and Allied Profession. IACAPAP Textbook of child and adolescent mental health. Available at: http://iacapap.org/iacapap-textbook-of-child-and-adolescent-mental-health. Accessed May 31, 2016.
25. American Academy of Child and Adolescent Psychiatry. Child and adolescent psychiatry resources for medical student educators. Available at: http://www.aacap.org/aacap/Resources_for_Primary_Care/CAP_Resources_for_Medical_Student_Educators.aspx. Accessed May 31, 2016.
26. Natt N, Dupras DM, Schultz HJ, et al. Impact of electronic faculty evaluation on resident return rates and faculty teaching performance. Med Teach 2006;28(2): e43–8.
27. Benjamin S, Robbins LI, Kung S. Online resources for assessment and evaluation. Acad Psychiatry 2006;30:498–504.
28. Reynolds K, Barnhill D, Sias J, et al. Use of the QR reader to provide real-time evaluation of residents' skills following surgical procedures. J Grad Med Educ 2014;6(4):738–41.
29. Havel LK, Powell SD, Cabaniss DL, et al. Smartphones, smart feedback: using mobile devices to collect in-the-moment feedback. Acad Psychiatry 2016. [Epub ahead of print].
30. Huang MP, Alessi NE. An informatics curriculum for psychiatry. Acad Psychiatry 1998;22:77–91.
31. Myers K, Cain S. Practice parameter for telepsychiatry with children and adolescents. J Am Acad Child Adolesc Psychiatry 2008;47(12):1468–83.
32. Sunderji N, Crawford A, Jovanovic M. Telepsychiatry in graduate medical education: a narrative review. Acad Psychiatry 2015;39(1):55–62.
33. Yellowlees PM, Odor A, Iosif AM, et al. Transcultural psychiatry made simple-asynchronous telepsychiatry as an approach to providing culturally relevant care. Telemed J E Health 2013;19(4):259–64.
34. Boston Children's Hospital. Center on Media and Child Health. Available at: http://cmch.tv/researchers/database-of-research/. Accessed May 31, 2016.

35. Ascherman LI, Rubin S. Current ethical issues in child and adolescent psycho-therapy. Child Adolesc Psychiatr Clin N Am 2008;17(1):21–35, vii–viii.
36. Thomas CR, Pastusek A. Boundary crossings and violations: time for child psychiatry to catch up. J Am Acad Child Adolesc Psychiatry 2012;51(9):858–60.
37. DeJong SM, Benjamin S, Meyer Anzia J, et al. Professionalism and the Internet in psychiatry: what to teach and how to teach it. Acad Psychiatry 2012;36(5): 356–62.
38. Gabbard GO, Kassaw KA, Perez-Garcia G. Professional boundaries in the era of the Internet. Acad Psychiatry 2011;35:168–74.
39. American Academy of Child and Adolescent Psychiatry. Health information technology and electronic medical records. Available at: http://www.aacap. org/aacap/clinical_practice_center/Business_of_Practice/Health_Information_Technology_and_Electronic_Medical_Records/Home.aspx. Accessed May 31, 2016.
40. Levine L, Waite BM, Bowman LL. Electronic media use, reading and academic distractibility in college youth. Cyberpsychol Behav 2007;10(4):560–6.
41. Levine LE, Waite BM, Bowman LL. Mobile media use, multitasking and distractibility. IJCBPL 2012;2(3):15–29.
42. Mueller PA, Oppenheimer DM. The pen is mightier than the keyboard: advantages of longhand over laptop note taking. Psychol Sci 2014;25(6):1159–68.
43. Shams L, Seitz AR. Benefits of multisensory learning. Trends Cogn Sci 2008; 12(11):411–7.
44. Mayer RE, Heiser J, Lonn S. Cognitive constraints on multimedia learning: when presenting more material results in less understanding. J Educ Psychol 2001; 93(1):187–98.
45. Barber LK, Santuzzi AM. Telepressure and college student employment: the costs of staying connected across social contexts. Stress Health 2016. [Epub ahead of print].
46. Nuutinen T, Roos E, Ray C, et al. Computer use, sleep duration and health symptoms: a cross-sectional study of 15-year olds in three countries. Int J Public Health 2014;59(4):619–28.
47. Chang AM, Aeschbach D, Duffy JE, et al. Evening use of light-emitting eReaders negatively affects sleep, circadian timing and next-morning alertness. Proc Natl Acad Sci U S A 2015;112(4):1232–7.

The Use of Health Information Technology Within Collaborative and Integrated Models of Child Psychiatry Practice

Sara Coffey, DO[a],*, Erik Vanderlip, MD, MPH[a], Barry Sarvet, MD[b]

KEYWORDS

- Integrated care • Health information technology • Child psychiatry
- Electronic health record • Collaborative care • Behavioral health clinician
- Child psychiatry access program

KEY POINTS

- There is a shortage of child and adolescent psychiatrists, even with increased recruitment of trainees traditional models of referral might not be able to meet the need.
- The behavioral health clinician model, child psychiatry access programs, and collaborative care have evidence to support improved access to care and quality of care.
- Integrated care models that are population focused, team-based, measurement-based, and evidenced-based are optimal to address treatment needs.
- Health information technology plays an important role in the delivery, accessibility, and quality of integrated practices.

INTRODUCTION

The Centers for Disease Control and Prevention reports a total of 13% to 20% of children living in the United States experience a mental disorder in a given year and the prevalence seems to be increasing.[1] The National Comorbidity Study of adolescents indicates that as many as 22% of adolescents aged 13 to 18 will have severe impairments.[2] However, studies show that in certain populations nearly 80% of children aged 6 to 17 years old do not receive mental health care.[3] There continues to be a

Disclosure Statement: The authors have nothing to disclose.
[a] Department of Psychiatry, Oklahoma State University School of Community Medicine, 4502 East 41st, Tulsa, OK 74135, USA; [b] Division of Child and Adolescent Psychiatry, Baystate Medical Center, 3300 Main Street 4th Floor, Springfield, MA 01199, USA
* Corresponding author.
E-mail address: Sara-coffey@ouhsc.edu

Child Adolesc Psychiatric Clin N Am 26 (2017) 105–115
http://dx.doi.org/10.1016/j.chc.2016.07.012   childpsych.theclinics.com
1056-4993/17/© 2016 Elsevier Inc. All rights reserved.

Abbreviations	
BHC	Behavioral health clinician
CCM	Collaborative care model
CPAP	Child psychiatry access program
EHR	Electronic health record
HIPPA	Health Information Portability Accountability Act
HIT	Health information technology
PCMH	Patient-centered medical home
PCP	Primary care physician
PHQ	Patient Health Questionnaire

shortage of child and adolescent psychiatrists and, although there has been an increase in the recruitment of child and adolescent psychiatry trainees, it is uncertain if these efforts alone will be sufficient to meet the needs of youth with mental illness.[4]

With this continued disparity of resources there is a need for both increased access and transformation in the delivery of care. In addition to an increase in the workforce, incorporating integrated care models into child and adolescent health is important. The Substance Abuse and Mental Health Services Administration defines integrated care as "the systematic coordination of general and behavioral healthcare," which includes mental health and substance abuse services under the larger umbrella of "behavioral health."[5] In child and adolescent psychiatry, integrated care models including the behavioral health clinician (BHC) integration in primary care model, the child psychiatry access programs (CPAP), and the collaborative care model (CCM) have shown promise in the care of pediatric patients.[6–8] These integrated delivery models go beyond colocated care and the patient-centered medical home (PCMH), which have also shown some promise in treatment of mental health conditions.[9] Regardless of the delivery system, it is vital providers communicate with each other and that care is population focused with a team approach using sound measurement and evidence to provide holistic care of children and adolescents.[10]

How health information technology (HIT) plays a role in these models is also of significance, because benefits and barriers exist across models. When HIT is used effectively it has the ability to improve upon care as usual and broaden access to specialist services. HIT can be described as, "the application of information processing involving both computer hardware and software that deals with the storage, retrieval, sharing, and use of health care information, data, and knowledge for communication and decision making."[11] Herein we look at how advancements in HIT can improve access and outcomes in the integrated care setting.

Integrated care is emerging as a compelling aspect of care delivery; however, defining what is meant by integrated care and the subsequent terms under its umbrella continues to be an issue. Some authors argue that further clarification of the definition of integrated care is in order.[12] With this is mind, we attempt to define the spectrum of care seen in pediatrics from care as usual to CCMs. Care as usual can be defined as a pediatrician seeing patients in an outpatient setting, referring the patient to mental health services when needed. In this model, the pediatrician and consulting child psychiatrist/mental health clinician might or might not communicate via phone and there may or may not be a shared medical record. This might be followed by the PCMH, which serves as a model of the organization of primary care. The PCMH incorporates certain core components, including comprehensive care, patient-centered care, coordinated care, accessible services, and quality and safety.[13] The American Academy of Pediatrics would add that the PCMH is compassionate, culturally competent, and family centered.[14] Colocated care can be described as a mental health specialist who is housed in the primary care clinic. Colocation is thought to improve access, streamline billing, and improve communication.[15]

For the purposes of this article, we look at 3 emerging methods of integrated care— the BHC, CPAP and CCM—as our models for integrated health care systems **(Table 1)**.[16–18] We then assess the potential for technology to improve communication, team-based care, evidence-based care, population management, and systematic tracking and quality improvement in each of the emerging integrated care models. CPAPs aim to improve access to care for children with mental health problems by providing primary care physicians (PCP) a collaborative relationship with regional child psychiatry teams. These teams offer consultation, care coordination, and educational programming.[7,19,20] In the Massachusetts Child Psychiatry Access Program model, telephone consultation serves as the primary interface between primary care clinicians and child psychiatrists and it is the most frequently used modality of service.[7,19] The BHC model includes the addition of a BHC (psychologist, social worker, nurse practitioner, or perhaps psychiatrist) who provides real-time collaboration and coordination with the BHC colocated in the primary care clinic. In the BHC model, a PCP would identify a patient in need of mental health services and during the appointment would request the BHC to see the patient in real time. The BHC could then evaluate the patient's emotional or behavioral health need and further collaborate with the PCP around treatment options. The BHC model lends itself to much variety both in the credentials of the BHC, as well as the time and scheduling within the primary care clinic.[21] The CCM is thought to operationalize the principals of the chronic care model in adults.[22,23] Bridging on the success in adult populations, further implementations in pediatric practice have been studied.[8] CCMs are team driven, led by a PCP with support from a care manager and consultation from a psychiatrist, who provides treatment recommendations for patients who are not achieving clinical goals. These goals are identified through ongoing review of a registry to manage a population of patients.[10]

With each iteration of health care delivery the added complexity and benefit of HIT becomes more apparent. HIT has the ability to enhance communication and care for our patients. Integrated platforms share further strengths and challenges; often there can be additional discrepancies between mental health and primary care professionals.[24,25] Some studies report that more than one-half of mental health providers' expressed concern around miscommunication with providers with the shared use of electronic health records.[26] Still other studies in primary care note providers indicating more burden than benefit with regard to e-health technologies.[24] Despite the challenges in HIT, there are certainly possibilities that HIT can benefit practices to become more population focused while enhancing measurement-based, team-based, and evidence-based care.

POPULATION-FOCUSED CARE: HEALTH INFORMATION TECHNOLOGY IN INTEGRATED CARE SETTINGS

Population-focused care incorporates an epidemiologic perspective while using evidence based practices to improve on the outcomes of the community.[27] CPAP models are population focused by nature, because often there is a state initiative to provide access to psychiatric consultation; for example, models like the Massachusetts Child Psychiatry Access Project are able to provide consultation and when indicated evaluation to multiple children and families across Massachusetts.[7,19,28] CPAP systems have the ability to understand the population through questions and concerns posed in consultation, the CPAP system can than tailor educational programming for pediatricians, which can be presented through web-based services including e-mail and central web sites.[19]

Table 1
Integrated care models in child and adolescent psychiatry

	Behavioral Health Clinician Model	Child Psychiatry Access Programs	Collaborative Care Model
Behavioral health team	On Site: behavioral health clinician: social worker, psychologist, nurse practitioner (rarely psychiatrist)	Off-site psychiatrist, therapist or care coordinator	On site: behavioral health care manager Off/on site: psychiatric consultant
Behavioral and primary care physicians work	In the same space, within the same facility, sharing health records	In separate facilities, health records are not typically shared	In the same space, within the same facility, sharing health records
Advantages in practice	Allows for collaboration of care, broad reach of the clinic population	Availability of immediacy of consultation, outreach of services (ability to reach more patients)	Measurable and definable, clinicians and teams can be held accountable to outcomes
Challenges in practice	Cultural changes in clinical practice, defaulting to colocation, limited ability for more structured and intensive behavioral health interventions or care coordination	System issues may limit collaboration, financing of services	Sustainability issues, limited studies in pediatric population, financing of services

In BHC models, initiating and maintaining a population based practice can be challenging. In the Advancing Care Together program, before the study BHC participants were not using data to track their populations and, although this changed with the implementation of the study, there continued to be barriers to using the electronic health record (EHR) to capture and share data between physical and mental health records. Often times behavioral health measures, like the Patient Health Questionnaire (PHQ)-9 were not captured routinely in discrete fields so that population data could be assessed. Additionally, programs that initially implemented population-focused measures had a difficult time maintaining them.[21,29]

BHC models have used a variety of interventions from tablets to personal digital assistants to acquire data for population management; however, staffing, compatibility of measures, and time leads to varying degrees of success, notably when information from personal electronic devices had to be entered manually into the EHR compliance decreased.[21,29,30] Yet some BHC practices use tablets that are directly transferable to the EHR. In those cases, BHCs were able to upload a variety of screening and monitoring measures, including the PHQ-9 and the Generalized Anxiety Disorder-7 that then transferred to the patient's electronic medical record.[29] Additionally, the EHR can be a useful tool to implement systemic protocols to assess patients for integrated care treatment; practices that implemented these systematic protocols have been seen to reach an average of 70% of their targeted population compared with an average of 7.9% in those that relied on clinician discretion.[29]

CCMs have used basic programs like Microsoft excel to track progress on PHQ-9s. Using a registry allowed the team to make treatment decisions based on reduction in PHQ-9 scores for the population as a whole.[8] Manual tracking with Excel spreadsheets is feasible, but often requires considerable staff time to maintain and do not integrate well within EHRs.[25] However, considerable opportunity exists for EHR-based registry development in the CCM.

TEAM-BASED CARE: HEALTH INFORMATION TECHNOLOGY IN INTEGRATED CARE SETTINGS

In integrated care models, team-based care includes primary care and mental health clinician(s) with clearly defined roles, who collaborate to ensure the best outcome for the patient.[18,21] In the BHC model, these teams are colocated. In the BHC model, HIT can be used to access scheduling and increase the dedicated time for collaboration, and when BHCs are not available for immediate consultation primary care clinicians can flag BHCs to follow-up with patients through the EHR.[21] What does seem to be a limitation to team-based care in the BHC model is the return to colocated care; often, BHCs initially available for consultation were relegated to seeing patients for individual services as the back-log for patient referrals grew.[21] In some BHC practices, the sharing and completion of encounter notes can be an issue.[21] The shared use of the EHR can allow for more consistent communication between primary care and mental health providers in the BHC model. How the clinical encounter note of the mental health clinician is documented might also pose additional challenges; because certain types of therapy notes (specifically process notes used for clinician reflection) have added Health Information Portability Accountability Act (HIPPA) regulations. Furthermore, federal regulations are undergoing change with regard to the limits of sharing confidential information for practitioners delivering and documenting care for substance abuse disorders.

CCMs have made modifications in the EHR to support integration; an electronic database allows team members to readily access data and make treatment decisions.[31] CCMs use team-based services through registries, which allow consulting psychiatrists and the care manager to review patients in real time in a collaborative way. Ideally, these registries should be accessible to each member of the team to ensure that everyone is on the same page.[10] Alerts and reminders within the EHR can notify team members in CCM to ensure appropriate follow-up.

CPAP models use e-mail to provide educational materials to the treating PCP in addition to providing consultation via telephone.[19] However, certain limitation persist in this model; often, interoperability between EHRs, HIPPA, and other factors limits the consulting psychiatrist's ability to view data. In some CPAP models, televideo supports can allow access to a child psychiatrist for further team collaboration and care.[20]

An innovative health home program in Oklahoma has given consumers iPads installed with the ability to Facetime therapist and/or crisis workers. These calls can then be discussed with a consulting psychiatrist or additional team members to make treatment decisions outside of clinic appointments.[32] What does seem to be important is the ability for practices to develop separate HIT interfaces programmed to extract specific data fields from EHRs and portable electronic devices that are bidirectional with the ability for team members to both enter and share data across platforms.[18,25]

MEASUREMENT-BASED CARE: HEALTH INFORMATION TECHNOLOGY IN INTEGRATED CARE SETTINGS

Measurement-based care uses clinical quantitative data closely correlated with disease state to monitor improvement.[33] HIT is playing an increasing role in the acquisition of this data, with self-monitoring devices, personal tracking devices (eg, glucometers), social media, and patient support web sites.[34] CCMs in adolescents have used a variety of evidenced-based mental health measures to monitor improvement in care including the PHQ-9, Screen for Child Anxiety Related Disorders (SCARED) anxiety inventory, the Columbia Impairment scale, and the Moods and Feelings Questionnaire. These measures can than be implemented into the EHR and exported to a registry for continued follow-up.[8,31] Integrating these measures into existing primary care models is important but can pose a challenge, because primary care–based EHRs often can lack the specific measurements used in behavioral health. Additionally, being able to use tablet devices to input patient data can pose a challenge with disparity of bidirectional systems.[18,25] Emerging mobile health technologies may be able to interface with the EHR and allow clinicians to more directly track their patients' clinical status, although these technologies have yet to receive full validation and are still in their infancy.

BHC also report using mental health measurements to assess a patients' severity of illness. However, in some instances this has been a challenge; often, the EHR in a primary care office does not capture mental health data in the way it would capture measurements pertinent to primary care.[29] Again the interoperability of these systems are key, because compliance decreases when measurements are taken on 1 system that are not directly transferable to the EHR.[21,29,30]

CPAPs have been noted to use claims data to track population-based outcomes. Using claims data allows for these programs to monitor their progress as function of the CPAP.[20] However, claims data are often limited in their ability to capture real-time data and lack a more accurate representation of health status.[32]

EVIDENCED BASED: HEALTH INFORMATION TECHNOLOGY IN INTEGRATED CARE SETTINGS

CCMs use EHRs and registries to monitor patients allowing consulting psychiatrists to make evidence-based treatment decisions based on diagnosis and symptom severity.[8,10,22,23,31] The registry is a shared document between the care manager, PCP, and consulting psychiatrist. The registry incorporates the existing tenants of integrated care, population-focused care, team-based care, and measurement-based care for the consulting psychiatrist to make evidenced-based decisions on the patients' shared information. Recommendations from the consulting psychiatrist can then be relayed through the EHR to the PCP, who will treat the patient accordingly.[10]

CPAP models use telephone or televideo to discuss diagnosis and treatment, allowing pediatricians access to a child and adolescent psychiatrist who will than provide evidenced-based recommendations in real time and can later fax the recommendations to the provider.[19,20] CPAP systems like the Partnership Access Line have a call database that uses information regarding diagnosis and treatment to confirm evidenced-based recommendations.[20] The use of telehealth technologies including a voice, image, or document delivery system can also lead to a better understanding of differences in care delivery between collaborators.[35]

BHC models have used tablets and other personal devices to acquire evidence-based mental health scales for patients.[29] This information could then be used to determine treatment options. However, BHC models typically do not include a consulting psychiatrist, so the psychopharmacology would be rendered by the PCP, who may or may not use the most up-to-date evidence. Additionally, depending on the referral of the patient or the availability of the BHC in practice the use of evidenced-based therapies might also be limited.[21]

SUMMARY

Each integrated model discussed herein has found innovative ways using HIT to improve patient care. HIT to support population-based care can be seen within all models, with CCMs using registries to track clinic populations, BHCs using the her to flag patients and clinicians, and CPAP models examining consultation questions to provide valuable education to participating providers.

With team-based care, we see the use of the EHR to allow interdisciplinary communication between providers, with similar challenges emerging between the bridging of primary care and mental health care records. Each model uses a variety of ways to connect behavioral health with primary care, from the EHR, to email to video conferencing, telephone and fax. Continued interoperability of these systems will likely improve the user's experience.

With regard to measurement-based care, the CCM and BHC models seem to be more effective, using evidence-based screening measures to track populations and communicate with providers. With CPAP's broad outreach, the focus can be more on educating individual clinicians about evidence-based screening tools available for PCPs. This ability to educate PCPs on a variety of screening tools, interventions, and treatment plans helps to improve a PCP's comfort in managing mental illness in children and in effect increases access to care.

The use of evidence-based medicine is seen in all 3 models. A distinction to be made between these models is the incorporation of a child psychiatrist as part of the treatment team in CCM and CPAP. Within the CCM and CPAP models, the use of evidenced-based care is essential in the delivery of care to patients. CPAP models have shown oversight to ensure recommendations made by consulting child psychiatrists are up to date and evidenced based, and CCM models also make use of evidenced-based algorithms to improve quality of care. Although BHC models likely rely on child psychiatrists as well, their incorporation into the team is variable. This potential disconnection might limit the ability for the PCP to feel confident in their psychopharmacology or have to rely on outside providers to manage the psychopharmacology of patient care. However, the ability to have a BHC co to help guide diagnosis and subsequent treatment decisions is certainly helpful to a primary care practice.

That being said, health care services are undergoing a rapid paradigm shift, with innovative and novel approaches to care delivery showing promise in line with ever-changing technology. HIT continues to enhance our experience, but is not without its challenges: staff buyin, upkeep, system crashes, user satisfaction, incompatible hardware, inability to upgrade software, and disruption in patient care during upgrades to name a few.[36] Integrated care models show success in adult medicine and ongoing work in pediatrics shows continued benefits. However, the sustainability and feasibility of these practice continues to be of some concern. HIT is a powerful resource to support these models in real time. HIT that supports integrated models to be population focused, team based, measurement based, and evidenced base are in even more demand. These delivery systems need to adapt to changes and integrate technology in a way that promotes rather than hinders care.

The sustainability of integrated care models is also of importance because staff time and clinician time not currently reimbursable can further impede full implementation of care. Specific challenges related to "the return to colocation" can be relieved with technological advances in scheduling. Access to data can be managed with patient-tracking devices. Interoperability of these systems continues to be of vital importance, because true collaboration insists on the ability to share information across forums.[25]

The Nationwide Health Information Network is also looking to advance standards and policies to ensure that patient information moves beyond a data acquisition tool to a collaborative effort where patients can own their health records and allow for the sharing of information between providers and practices.[37] The use of health information exchanges to close this "data loop" can be instrumental in the bidirectionality of data. Advances including decision support tools within the EHR indicating when screening is needed is also of value in integrated models.[18] Additionally, the use of the EHR to tailor medication dosages and adherence to medication is another feature that integrated practices could potentially benefit from.[38]

Barriers related to sharing mental health records remains, with further restrictions related to HIPPA and mental health providers' beliefs and implementation of EHRs.[39,40] What is more, a national study by the Center for Studying Health System Change notes that both primary care and psychiatrist were behind other specialist in using HIT to access notes and exchange data with other clinicians. Delay in implementation is likely multifactorial, because practice size can often dictate implementation of EHRs and psychiatric practices more likely to be small.[41] However, continued issues around privacy likely persist as well, with mental health clinicians reporting concerns with confidentiality of mental health records.[42] Additionally, patients with "sensitive" information in their medical record, mental health, substance abuse, and so on, might choose to restrict these data from being shared with providers, which could limit collaboration.[43,44] Additional barriers including payment structures continues to be an impediment in these services as well.[45] However, leadership that can be forward thinking, willing to take on risks and learn from previous implementations with a data-driven approach has the potential to be successful implementing these innovative practices.[18]

REFERENCES

1. Perou R. Mental health surveillance among children — United States, 2005–2011. Atlanta, GA: Centers for Disease Control and Prevention; 2013. Available

at: http://www.cdc.gov/mmwr/preview/mmwrhtml/su6202a1.htm?viewtype= print. Accessed April 25, 2016.

2. Merikangas KR, He J, Burstein M, et al. Lifetime Prevalence of mental disorders in US adolescents: results from the national comorbidity study-adolescent supplement (NCS-A). J Am Acad Child Adolesc Psychiatry 2010; 49(10):980–9.

3. Kataoka SH, Zhang L, Wells KB. Unmet need for mental health care among U.S. children: variation by ethnicity and insurance status. Am J Psychiatry 2002;159(9):1548–55.

4. Thomas CR, Holzer CE. The Continuing shortage of child and adolescent psychiatrists. J Am Acad Child Adolesc Psychiatry 2006;45(9):1023–31.

5. SAMHSA-HRSA Center for Integrated Health Solutions. What is integrated care. SAMHSA-HRSA. Available at: http://www.integration.samhsa.gov/about-us/what-is-integrated-care. Accessed April 27, 2016.

6. Cohen DJ, Davis M, Balasubramanian BA, et al. Integrating behavioral health and primary care: consulting, coordinating and collaborating among professionals. J Am Board Fam Med 2015;28(Supplement 1):S21–31.

7. Sarvet B, Gold J, Bostic JQ, et al. Improving access to mental health care for children: the Massachusetts child psychiatry access project. Pediatrics 2010;126(6): 1191–200.

8. Richardson LP, Ludman E, McCauley E, et al. Collaborative care for adolescents with depression in primary care: a randomized clinical trial. JAMA 2014;312(8): 809–16.

9. Toomey SL, Chan E, Ratner JA, et al. The patient-centered medical home, practice patterns, and functional outcomes for children with attention deficit/hyperactivity disorder. Acad Pediatr 2011;11(6):500–7.

10. American Psychiatric Association. Dissemination of integrated care within adult primary care settings: The collaborative care model. The Collaborative Care Model. Available at: https://www.psychiatry.org/psychiatrists/practice/professional-interests/integrated-care/collaborative-care-model. Accessed May 20, 2016.

11. US Department of Health and Human Services, Health Information Technology. What is Health IT? Available at: http://www.hrsa.gov/healthit/toolbox/oralhealthittoolbox/introduction/whatishealthit.html. Accessed May 4, 2016.

12. Singer SJ, Burgers J, Friedberg M, et al. Defining and measuring integrated patient care: promoting the next frontier in health care delivery. Med Care Res Rev 2010;68(1):112–27.

13. Agency for Healthcare Research and Quality. Defining the PCMH. Available at: https://pcmh.ahrq.gov/page/defining-pcmh. Accessed April 27, 2016.

14. Dickens M, Green J, Kohrt A, et al. American Academy of Pediatrics: the medical home. Pediatrics 1992;90(5):774. Available at: http://pediatrics.aappublications.org/content/pediatrics/90/5/774.full.pdf. Accessed May 20, 2016.

15. American Academy of Child and Adolescent Psychiatry (AACAP). A guide to building collaborative mental health care partnerships In Pediatric primary care. 2010. Available at: https://www.aacap.org/App_Themes/AACAP/docs/clinical_practice_center/guide_to_building_collaborative_mental_health_care_partnerships.pdf. Accessed April 30, 2016.

16. Heath B, Wise Romero P, Reynolds KA. Review and proposed standard framework for levels of integrated healthcare. Washington, DC: SAMHSA-HRSA Center for Integrated Health Solutions; 2013.

17. AIMS Center Newsletter: Stepped Model of Integrated Health Care. 2016. Available at: https://aims.uw.edu/stepped-model-integrated-behavioral-health care?utm_source=AIMS+Center+Newsletter&utm_campaign=4e1004dc9c-AIMSCenter Newsletter_April-May_2015&utm_medium=email&utm_term=0_5e264f9d0f-4e1004dc9c-294081313. Accessed May 12, 2016.

18. Cohen DJ, Davis MM, Hall JD, et al. Guidebook of professional practices for behavioral health and primary care integration: observations from exemplary sites. Rockville (MD): Agency for Healthcare Research and Quality; 2015. Available at: http://integrationacademy.ahrq.gov/sites/default/files/AHRQ_Academy Guidebook.pdf. Accessed May 17, 2016.

19. Sarvet B, Gold J, Straus JH. Bridging the divide between child psychiatry and primary care: the use of telephone consultation within a population-based collaborative system. Child Adolesc Psychiatr Clin N Am 2011;20(1):41–53.

20. Hilt RJ, Romaire MA, McDonell MG, et al. The partnership access line: evaluating a child psychiatry consult program in Washington state. JAMA Pediatr 2013;167(2):162–8.

21. Davis MM, Balasubramanian BA, Cifuentes M, et al. Clinician staffing, scheduling, and engagement strategies among primary care practices delivering integrated care. J Am Board Fam Med 2015;28(Supplement 1):S32–40.

22. Katon W, Von Korff M, Lin E, et al. "Collaborative management to achieve depression treatment guidelines. JAMA 1995;273(13):1026–31.

23. Katon W, Robinson P, Von Korff M, et al. A multifaceted intervention to improve treatment of depression in primary care. Arch Gen Psychiatry 1996;53(10):924–32. Available at: http://www.ncbi.nlm.nih.gov/pubmed/8857869.

24. Aultman JM, Dean E. Beyond privacy: benefits and burdens of e-health technologies in primary care. J Clin Ethics 2014;25(1):50–64.

25. Cifuentes M, Davis M, Gunn R, et al. Electronic health record challenges, workarounds, and solutions observed in practices integrating behavioral health and primary care. J Am Board Fam Med 2015;28:S63–72.

26. Shank N, Willborn E, Pytlikzillig L, et al. Electronic health records: eliciting behavioral health providers' beliefs. Community Ment Health J 2011;48(2):249–54.

27. Ibrahim MA, Savitz LA, Carey TS, et al. Population-based health principles in medical and public health practice. J Public Health Manag Pract 2001;7(3):75–81.

28. Gabel S. The integration of mental health into pediatric practice: pediatricians and child and adolescent psychiatrists working together in new models of care. J Pediatr 2010;157(5):848–51.

29. Balasubramanian BA, Fernald D, Dickinson LM, et al. REACH of interventions integrating primary care and behavioral health. J Am Board Fam Med 2015;28(Supplement 1):S71–85.

30. Cohen DJ, Balasubramanian BA, Isaacson NF, et al. Coordination of health behavior counseling in primary care. Ann Fam Med 2011;9:406–15.

31. Richardson L, Mccauley E, Katon W. Collaborative care for adolescent depression: a pilot study. Gen Hosp Psychiatry 2009;31(1):36–45.

32. Vanderlip, E Improving access and quality of children's mental health treatments. Presented at the Oklahoma Department of Mental Health and Substance Abuse, Children's Behavioral Health Conference. Norman, Oklahoma, May 12, 2016.

33. Kerr E, Krein SL, Vijan S, et al. Avoiding pitfalls in chronic disease quality measurement: a case for the next generation of technical quality measures. Am J Manag Care 2001;7(11):1033–43.

34. Brennan PF, Valdez R, Alexander G, et al. Patient-centered care, collaboration, communication, and coordination: a report from AMIA's 2013 Policy Meeting. J Am Med Inform Assoc 2015;22(e1):e2–6.
35. Shih FJ, Shih FJ, Pan Y, et al. Dilemma of applying telehealth for overseas organ transplantation: comparison on perspectives of health professionals and e-health information and communication technologists in Taiwan. Transplant Proc 2014; 46(4):1019–21.
36. George S, Garth B, Fish A, et al. Factors shaping effective utilization of health information technology in urban safety-net clinics. Health Informatics J 2013;19(3): 183–97.
37. HealthIT.gov. Nationwide Health Information Network. Available at: https://www.healthit.gov/policy-researchers-implementers/nationwide-health-information-network-nwhin. Accessed May 11, 2016.
38. Dorr D, Bonner LM, Cohen AN, et al. Informatics systems to promote improved care for chronic illness: a literature review. J Am Med Inform Assoc 2007; 14(2):156.
39. Fetter M. Personal health records: protecting behavioral health consumers' rights. Issues Ment Health Nurs 2009;30(11):720–2.
40. Mcgregor B, Mack D, Wrenn G, et al. Improving service coordination and reducing mental health disparities through adoption of electronic health records. Psychiatr Serv 2015;66(9):985–7.
41. Wolfe J. Few psychiatrists take advantage of Medicare EHR incentives. Psychiatr News 2013;48(24):1.
42. Salomon RM, Blackford JU, Rosenbloom ST, et al. Openness of patients' reporting with use of electronic records: psychiatric clinicians' views. J Am Med Inform Assoc 2010;17(1):54–60.
43. Leventhal JC, Cummins JA, Schwartz PH, et al. Designing a system for patients controlling providers' access to their electronic health records: organizational and technical challenges. J Gen Intern Med 2014;30(S1):17–24.
44. Tierney WM, Alpert SA, Byrket A, et al. Provider responses to patients controlling access to their electronic health records: a prospective cohort study in primary care. J Gen Intern Med 2014;30(S1):31–7.
45. Floyd P. Integrating physical and behavioral health a major step toward population health management. Westchester, IL: Healthcare Financial Management; 2016. p. 64–71.

Confidentiality and Privacy for Smartphone Applications in Child and Adolescent Psychiatry

Unmet Needs and Practical Solutions

Emily Wu, MD[a,b],*, John Torous, MD[b,c], Rashad Hardaway, MD[d],
Thomas Gutheil, MD[b]

KEYWORDS

• Technology • Smartphones • Privacy • Security • Confidently

KEY POINTS

- Confidentiality and privacy are critical in child and adolescent psychiatry and necessary for digital tools like smartphone applications (apps) to maintain if they are to be useful clinical tools in the future.
- Currently little is known about the confidentiality and privacy of digital tools like smartphone apps for clinical care.
- Important issues to consider include disclosure of information sharing, access privilege, privacy and trust, risk and benefit analysis, and the need for standardization.
- Child and adolescent psychiatrists need to stay up to date on privacy, security, and confidentiality of digital technologies in order help patients and parents make informed decisions and shape the next generation of these tools.

INTRODUCTION

As digital technologies like computers and smartphones become increasingly pervasive, their potential to advance health care has been well recognized. Electronic medical records are now ubiquitous in many clinical practices, although their use remains lower in psychiatry than in other medical specialties.[1] This slower adoption

Disclosures: None.
[a] Harvard Longwood Psychiatry Residency Training Program, Harvard Medical School, 330 Brookline Avenue, Rabb-2, Boston, MA 02115, USA; [b] Department of Psychiatry, Beth Israel Deaconess Medical Center, Harvard Medical School, 330 Brookline Avenue, Boston, MA 02115, USA; [c] Division of Clinical Informatics, Beth Israel Deaconess Medical Center, Harvard Medical School, 1330 Beacon Street, Suite 400, Brookline, MA 02446, USA; [d] Department of Psychiatry and Behavioral Medicine, Seattle Children's Hospital, 4800 Sand Point Way NE, Seattle, WA 98105, USA
* Corresponding author. 330 Brookline Avenue, Rabb 2, Boston, MA 02115.
E-mail address: ewu4@bidmc.harvard.edu

Child Adolesc Psychiatric Clin N Am 26 (2017) 117–124
http://dx.doi.org/10.1016/j.chc.2016.07.006
1056-4993/17/© 2016 Elsevier Inc. All rights reserved.

of technology stands in contrast to how younger individuals today are embracing smartphone technology. The latest national survey 2 years ago indicated that, in 2014, 73% of teenagers in the United States owned a smartphone.[2] Today smartphone technology is widely adopted by teenagers and children for accessing social media, playing games, and browsing the Internet. Although smartphones are not yet widely used toward promoting mental health, the potential of smartphone applications (apps) to bring new real-time data, responsive monitoring, and even adjunctive therapeutic tools to child and adolescent psychiatry has been increasingly recognized. Today, even social media services like Facebook will flag posts concerning for self-harm[3]; mood-monitoring apps can track depressive symptoms[4]; and a plethora of apps offer self-help and therapy services from the convenience of the phone.[5]

Recent research suggests numerous potential uses of new smartphone technologies for clinical care in child and adolescent technology. Although beyond the scope of this article, studies have already shown the potential of smartphones to assist in delivering cognitive behavioral therapy in the treatment of anxiety for children[6] and in helping children better cope with pain.[7] Other researchers are investigating how smartphones can help adolescent patients report symptoms with less recall bias.[8,9] However, in order to be useful clinical tools, smartphone apps have to demonstrate not only that they can capture useful information but also that they are safe to use, respect patient privacy, maintain confidentiality, comply with both local and federal guidelines, and meet the field's professional and ethical standards. Yet in many cases, new technologies like smartphone apps have advanced more rapidly than health care regulations and professional society guidelines, creating a need for better education and action by the health care system.[10] Thus, the aim of this article is to offer a summary of current knowledge, practices, and existing gaps regarding confidentiality and privacy for mobile devices when offering child and adolescent psychiatric services and to provide a discussion on how the field can respond to this new challenge by establishing best practices and useful guidelines. Given the nascent nature of this topic and the dynamic pace of technology, the authors do not intend this article to be a comprehensive review but rather a guided discussion highlighting salient topics.

STAKEHOLDERS

Currently, there is a lack of data regarding the level of understanding and consensus on privacy laws and clinical practice approaches on medical technology adoption. A 2012 survey of parents' knowledge and opinions about health care laws regarding technology to facilitate communication between pediatricians and youth revealed that only one-third approved of technology for communication between their children and pediatricians and nearly half were unaware that adolescents could receive confidential sexuality-related information without parental permission.[11] Since this study was conducted in 2012, smartphones have become more prevalent and heath information Web sites more common. Parental opinion should again be assessed in a now even more digital and connected world, where youth are using technology not only to contact their clinicians about health information but also to access health information via chat rooms, Internet forums, numerous Web sites, and smartphone apps.

In addition, clinicians must be educated and ensure they are up to date on privacy and confidentiality regulations for child and adolescent patients. Although professional guidelines, such as the American Psychiatric Associations' Principles of Medical Ethics, underscore the importance of safeguarding patient confidences and privacy,[12] such guidelines do not offer concrete advice in an evolving digital health landscape. A recent survey study of 650 clinicians at an academic medical center, regarding their comfort addressing sexual and mental health issues, revealed that only slightly more than half could correctly answer questions on legal knowledge regarding confidentiality and consent related to these topics. Seventy-six percent of clinicians who partook in the study noted they thought they needed further education and training regarding these regulations and guidelines.[13] Although this study did not assess clinicians' familiarity with delivering care via digital devices or telepsychiatry platforms, it is likely there would be even greater levels of uncertainty regarding confidentiality and consent, given that such tools are nascent in the field. Further data are needed regarding what child and adolescent psychiatrists understand and know about consent and confidentiality when using digital tools.

Moreover, few national guidelines offer tangible advice. Considering health records, where more regulation and guidance exist, the Agency for Health Quality and Research in 2015 released a technical brief entitled "Core Functionality in Pediatric Health Records"; this brief indirectly offers some guidance in considering regulations for digital technologies aimed at child and adolescent patients. Regarding electronic health records (EHRs), the report notes "privacy requirements may vary by age and permission levels, [and] may vary based on clinical role or family relationship, thus complicating universal standards or guidelines."[14] The report notes that a robust privacy infrastructure is critical to the success of EHRs and that it is important that privacy revolves around patients. Yet, the report also brings up the complexities of maintaining digital privacy and granting access to information to groups, such as stepparents, foster care providers, and guardians and in situations such as when child abuse is suspected.[14] Although the report does not discuss smartphone apps, it clearly outlines important points that clinicians, patients, family members, and technology developers alike must be mindful of when considering mobile technologies for clinical care.

It is also necessary to consider the patients' perspective regarding confidentiality and consent in using digital technologies for mental heath care. Although few studies have specifically focused on the perspective and knowledge of child and adolescent psychiatry patients on this important topic, some have indirectly addressed the issue and provided early data. A study of 521 youths, aged 17 to 24 years, in Canada noted that most have turned to the Internet to learn about mental health and that 87% view privacy as very important when using online tools.[15] However, data are lacking on how valuing online privacy translates into online actions; studies are needed to illuminate how children and adolescents are actually using mobile and online tools related to psychiatry. Many users may not realize that most smartphone apps and Web sites fall outside of the scope of the Health Insurance Portability and Accountability Act (HIPAA); thus, the health information they provide to such services may be sold, marketed, and traded without their control.[16] Indeed, this problem, essentially a lack of informed consent for patients, is a fundamental flaw in HIPAA.

Among parents, clinicians, and child and adolescent patients, as well as even in national guidelines, clear guidance and robust knowledge are lacking regarding confidentiality and consent for new mobile tools like smartphones. For any regulatory and education system to work effectively, there must be agreement and understanding among all stakeholders; this will be an important endeavor going forward. An important first step will be undertaking research to better assess the current knowledge of all stakeholders and to identify immediate targets for educational interventions. Although such efforts will need to be customized to each stakeholder and population, later the authors discuss several aspects to consider when addressing issues of confidentiality and consent for mobile tools used in child and adolescent psychiatry.

ISSUES TO CONSIDER
Disclosure

Although an app can be downloaded and used anywhere, the health care laws regarding disclosure of adolescents' mental health records to parents and legal guardians vary from state to state. Even with electronic medical records, it is complicated to determine when and if parents can access mental health information. In some states, parents and guardians are permitted to access the mental health records of minors.[17] In response, the American Academy of Child and Adolescent Psychiatry proposed a 2012 policy statement requesting disclosure to both patients and family members regarding the scope of care and the information that will and can be shared with family members or other health care providers.[18] Providing a similar disclosure about who will be able to access data from a mental health app is an important point to consider, requiring discussion among clinicians, patients, and family members. This discussion is especially important, as studies suggest that parents are usually uncertain about their children receiving confidential care,[19,20] although those with higher trust toward their child's physician tend to be more comfortable with the child receiving these confidential services.[19] Another case that must be considered is disclosure in the setting of emergencies. Individuals may report symptoms indicating the high risk of self-harm or suicide; thus, because emergencies are exceptions to confidentiality, it is important for all involved parties to know the following: what are the thresholds or types of entered data that may potentially activate an emergency response system? In a related context, if app data are going to be monitored by a clinician, the frequency and schedule of such monitoring should be made clear. Finally, all parties need to be aware that unintended disclosure may happen if a patient is observed using the app or leaves the app running on the phone in a public place.

Access Privilege

Laws in all 50 states and the District of Columbia allow adolescents to receive certain health care services without parental consent.[21] However, the age of consent required for mental health services varies from state to state. Health information technologies like smartphone apps must be designed to reinforce confidentiality in protecting adolescents' rights to seek mental health services. New digital health care tools should be designed with different levels of access, in order to restrict sharing of confidential health information, such as psychological assessments, risk factor screening, or substance treatment, with parents or guardians. Likewise, it is also important to have the functionality present that would allow the parents the option of keeping sensitive family histories confidential from their children, such as those involving Huntington disease, Lynch syndrome, human immunodeficiency virus, or psychiatric illness. Given that most states require some form of parental or guardian consent at least to initiate mental health services, technology platforms should be developed to reinforce identity proofing and authentication of parents and patients. Carefully designed login procedures and protocols will be necessary to ensure confidentiality is maintained.[14,22] Some studies have used color-coded screen backgrounds to highlight confidential elements in patients' electronic record to achieve clear delineation.[23] In addition to access, sociocultural factors should also be taken into account for designing different interfaces and different language options for patients and families.[24] Other studies have used a hybrid cloud structure to reinforce the access control policy, which allows different types of users to gain different access privileges within the same digital health care record.[25] Bourgeois and colleagues[26] suggest implementing an access control policy based on patients' age; they have piloted a hybrid approach toward control of medical data with a pediatric and adolescent personally controlled health record platform called Indivo.

Privacy and Trust

Beyond authentication and login procedures, technology platforms like smartphone apps must maintain user trust by keeping health data secure and private. In order to ensure security and privacy, there are 2 separate but related factors that must be considered: transparency and data security.

Data security refers to how a technology platform protects information it collects and transmits. Although the federal privacy law, HIPAA, mandates certain levels of data security through encryption, many apps fall outside of the scope of HIPAA, which means that many apps are not mandated to secure the health data they collect or transmit.[27] The scope of the problem was highlighted in October 2015 when researchers examined 79 health apps on the British National Health Services App Library. They found that none of them encrypted data on the device; 35 transmitted personally identifiable data over the Internet, and only one-third encrypted data during wireless transmission.[28] An industry report by the company Arxan noted that 86% of the health apps approved by the US Food and Drug Administration that they tested did not adequately address at least 2 of the top 10 Open Web Application Security Project risks.[29] To build the trust necessary for patients to provide their mental health data, apps will have to improve their security standards and prove they can safely secure personal health data.

But trust goes beyond just security, as an app can have world-class security but also sell patient health data and mental health information. All apps should have privacy policies that outline if patient data will be sold, traded, or marketed; it is important to understand such before considering any health app. Although there have been no studies focusing on the privacy policies of mental health apps aimed toward children and adolescents, research in the area of general mental health apps suggests that many apps operate under a business model of collecting personal mental health data and then selling such for a profit to data brokers.[16] Updated privacy laws on deidentified data, recording and transmitting data, increased public awareness, and regular security enhancements[10] are needed.

Even if apps are secure and transparent, there remains a risk of confidentiality breaches during the process surrounding their use in the health care setting. In a recent article, Dufendach and colleagues[14] listed many potential points for breaches of confidentiality via electronic tools, including releasing sensitive laboratory results, automated posting of an explanation of benefits, issuing after-visit summaries, and requesting copies of medical records. Although most physicians are confident in discussing sensitive issues with adolescent patients and think that adolescents should be assured of access to confidential care, they also think there are many existing barriers to providing such care.[13] For example, insurance usually requires explanation of benefits, with an itemized list of services received sent to parents. Likewise, the electronic medical record usually prints out an after-visit summary, including itemized problem lists, tests, and medications. This summary may also consequently disclose the confidential health information to the parents or guardians. Thus, psychiatrists should receive adequate training to understand how electronic tools, such as apps, will fit into the clinical structure and how information from them may be shared in the clinical environment.[13]

Risk/Benefit Analysis

Using a mental health app involves a decision of weighing the potential risks versus potential benefits. As outlined earlier, poor security and lack of transparency are common in many apps and present a clear risk to patients. This problem directly hinders utilization of digital platforms like smartphone apps.[30] On the other hand, efficacy data are lacking regarding apps for child and adolescent psychiatry[31]; this lack makes it difficult to understand the clinical benefits of many apps. More clinical data on apps will be necessary to help move the risk/benefit ratio for app usage in child and adolescent psychiatry. Thus, it will be important for child and adolescent psychiatrists to stay up to date on the research evidence and industry claims in order to guide both their patients and parents through an informed discussion on the current risks and benefits of app use. It will also be necessary to increase health technology literacy among parents, so that they better understand the risks and benefits of various platforms and can make informed decisions.[13]

Need for Standards

Standards are needed across various health technology platforms to not only make it easier to evaluate and understand how these platforms work but also to support interoperability. The Council on Clinical Information Technology, American Academy of Pediatrics,[32] has proposed that the development of adolescent health portals must include universal standards for content, information assurance, and data exchange that meet adolescents' health needs. In addition to standards, psychiatrists must work with technology developers to ensure that data-exchange standards provide accurate data transmission and reception, accurate data interpretation, and data presentation in the correct user interfaces. Psychiatrists must also begin to investigate apps and help create standards and ratings for which apps may be useful in clinical care and which may be dangerous.[33,34] Having libraries of apps that child and adolescent psychiatrists have thoroughly studied and feel comfortable recommending will ensure that patients are receiving useful and safe apps. Technology companies and vendors can also help by offering clear on-screen labeling of confidential data elements and making privacy policies more readable and easier to understand.[23]

SUMMARY

Although smartphone use for child and adolescent psychiatry offers the potential of new diagnostic tools and adjunctive therapeutic interventions, these devices are not yet first-line clinical tools. Considering how many youths now own and regularly use smartphones, there will likely be greater momentum to explore the clinical evidence base to determine whether apps and connected sensors have useful roles in clinical care for child and adolescent psychiatry patients. But beyond evidence of efficacy, there is also an unmet need in regard to the privacy and confidentiality capabilities, as well as standards, of smartphone apps for child and adolescent psychiatry. If clinicians, parents, and patients all lack confidence in apps' ability to protect mental health information, then the foundation of trust will remain lacking and the clinical potential of these new tools will not be achievable. Although there is currently a lack of knowledge and experience regarding privacy and confidentiality of smartphone technology for child and adolescent psychiatry, a focus on education, access privilege, data security, transparency, and national standards is a positive first step to consider.

REFERENCES

1. Kokkonen EW, Davis SA, Lin HC, et al. Use of electronic medical records differs by specialty and office settings. J Am Med Inform Assoc 2013;20(e1):e33–8.

2. Lenhart A. A majority of American teens report access to a computer, game console, smartphone and a tablet. Pew Research Center. 2015. Available at: http://www.pewinternet.org/2015/04/09/a-majority-of-american-teens-report-access-to-a-computer-game-console-smartphone-and-a-tablet/. Accessed April 21, 2016.
3. Facebook introduces new tools to help prevent suicide. NBC News. 2015. Available at: http://www.nbcnews.com/tech/social-media/facebook-introduces-new-tools-help-prevent-suicide-n313546. Accessed April 22, 2016.
4. Torous J, Staples P, Shanahan M, et al. Utilizing a personal smartphone custom app to assess the patient health questionnaire-9 (PHQ-9) depressive symptoms in patients with major depressive disorder. JMIR Ment Health 2015;2(1):e8.
5. Karasouli E, Adams A. Assessing the evidence for e-resources for mental health self-management: a systematic literature review. JMIR Ment Health 2014;1(1):e3.
6. Pramana G, Parmanto B, Kendall PC, et al. The SmartCAT: an m-health platform for ecological momentary intervention in child anxiety treatment. Telemed J E Health 2014;20(5):419–27.
7. Schatz J, Schlenz AM, Mcclellan CB, et al. Changes in coping, pain, and activity after cognitive-behavioral training: a randomized clinical trial for pediatric sickle cell disease using smartphones. Clin J Pain 2015;31(6):536–47.
8. Kolar DR, Bürger A, Hammerle F, et al. Aversive tension of adolescents with anorexia nervosa in daily course: a case-controlled and smartphone-based ambulatory monitoring trial. BMJ Open 2014;4(4):e004703.
9. Könen T, Dirk J, Schmiedek F. Cognitive benefits of last night's sleep: daily variations in children's sleep behavior are related to working memory fluctuations. J Child Psychol Psychiatry 2015;56(2):171–82.
10. Mamlin BW, Tierney WM. The promise of information and communication technology in healthcare: extracting value from the chaos. Am J Med Sci 2016;351(1):59–68.
11. Thompson LA, Martinko T, Budd P, et al. Meaningful use of a confidential adolescent patient portal. J Adolesc Health 2016;58(2):134–40.
12. APA Committee on Confidentiality. Guidelines on confidentiality. Am J Psychiatry 1987;144(11):1522.
13. Riley M, Ahmed S, Reed BD, et al. Physician knowledge and attitudes around confidential care for minor patients. J Pediatr Adolesc Gynecol 2015;28(4):234–9.
14. Dufendach K, Eichenberher J, McPhetters M, et al. Core functionality in pediatric electronic health records. 2015. Available at: https://www.effectivehealthcare.ahrq.gov/ehc/products/591/2070/pediatric-EHR-report-150417.pdf. Accessed April 26, 2016.
15. Wetterlin FM, Mar MY, Neilson EK, et al. eMental health experiences and expectations: a survey of youths' Web-based resource preferences in Canada. J Med Internet Res 2014;16(12):e293.
16. Glenn T, Monteith S. Privacy in the digital world: medical and health data outside of HIPAA protections. Curr Psychiatry Rep 2014;16(11):494.
17. Houston M. The psychiatric medical record, HIPAA, and the use of electronic medical records. Child Adolesc Psychiatr Clin N Am 2010;19(1):107–14.
18. Confidentiality in health information technology. 2012. Available at: http://www.aacap.org/aacap/policy_statements/2012/Confidentiality_in_Health_Information_Technology.aspx. Accessed May 15, 2016.
19. Sasse RA, Aroni RA, Sawyer SM, et al. Confidential consultations with adolescents: an exploration of Australian parents' perspectives. J Adolesc Health 2013;52:786.

20. Tebb K, Karime Hernandez L, Shafer M, et al. Understanding the attitudes of Latino parents toward confidential health services for teens. J Adolesc Health 2012;50:572.
21. Giannone G. Computer-supported weight-based drug infusion concentrations in the neonatal intensive care unit. Comput Inform Nurs 2005;23(2):100–5.
22. Sittig DF, Singh H. Legal, ethical, and financial dilemmas in electronic health record adoption and use. Pediatrics 2011;127(4):e1042–7.
23. Anoshiravani A, Gaskin GL, Groshek MR, et al. Special requirements for electronic medical records in adolescent medicine. J Adolesc Health 2012;51(5):409–14.
24. Brown SM, Aboumatar HJ, Francis L, et al, Privacy, Access, and Engagement Task Force of the Libretto Consortium of the Gordon and Betty Moore Foundation. Balancing digital information-sharing and patient privacy when engaging families in the intensive care unit. J Am Med Inform Assoc 2016. [Epub ahead of print].
25. Rezaeibagha F, Mu Y. Distributed clinical data sharing via dynamic access-control policy transformation. Int J Med Inform 2016;89:25–31.
26. Bourgeois FC, Taylor PL, Emans SJ, et al. Whose personal control? Creating private, personally controlled health records for pediatric and adolescent patients. J Am Med Inform Assoc 2008;15(6):737–43.
27. Blenner SR, Köllmer M, Rouse AJ, et al. Privacy policies of android diabetes apps and sharing of health information. JAMA 2016;315(10):1051–2.
28. Huckvale K, Prieto JT, Tilney M, et al. Unaddressed privacy risks in accredited health and wellness apps: a cross-sectional systematic assessment. BMC Med 2015;13:214.
29. 5th annual state of application security report. Arxan. Available at: https://www.arxan.com/wp content/uploads/2016/01/State_of_Application_Security_2016_Healthcare_Report.pdf. Accessed May 2, 2016.
30. Li H, Wu J, Gao Y, et al. Examining individuals' adoption of healthcare wearable devices: an empirical study from privacy calculus perspective. Int J Med Inform 2016;88:8–17.
31. Wu E, Torous J, Harper G. A gap in the literature: clinical role for smartphone applications for depression care among adolescents? J Am Acad Child Adolesc Psychiatry 2016;55(7):630–1.
32. Council on Clinical Information Technology. Policy statement-using personal health records to improve the quality of health care for children. Pediatrics 2009;124(1):403–9.
33. Chan S, Torous J, Hinton L, et al. Towards a framework for evaluating mobile mental health apps. Telemed J E Health 2015;21(12):1038–41.
34. Torous JB, Chan SR, Yellowlees PM, et al. To use or not? Evaluating ASPECTS of smartphone apps and mobile technology for clinical care in psychiatry. J Clin Psychiatry 2016;77(6):e734–8.

The Economic Benefits of Mobile Apps for Mental Health and Telepsychiatry Services When Used by Adolescents

Adam C. Powell, PhD[a],*, Milton Chen, PhD[b],
Chanida Thammachart, MA[c],1

KEYWORDS

- Return on investment • Telemedicine • Telepsychiatry • mHealth
- Mobile applications

KEY POINTS

- Mobile applications for mental health and telepsychiatry provide both direct and indirect benefits.
- Digital tools for mental health positively impact patients, caregivers, and clinicians.
- A common framework of questions can be used to evaluate return on investment, regardless of the nature of the service or tool under consideration.

BACKGROUND

According to a 2015 Pew Research Center poll, 73% of teens have access to a smartphone, 58% have access to a tablet, and 87% have access to a computer.[1] Among early teens, smartphone use is also high, with 64% of boys and 72% of girls age 13 to 14 years having access. Although smartphone use is more common in high-income households, 61% of teens in households earning less than $30,000 per year have access to a smartphone. Traditional racial disparities in access are reversed for smartphones, as 85% of non-Hispanic black teens have access, compared with 71% of non-Hispanic white teens and 71% of Hispanic teens. Smartphone ownership is common among people with mental health conditions, with one study finding an

Disclosures: See last page of article.
[a] Payer+Provider Syndicate, 111 Beach Street 4E, Boston, MA 02111, USA; [b] VSee, 3188 Kimlee Drive, San Jose, CA 95132, USA; [c] University of New England, 11 Hills Beach Road, Biddeford, ME 04005, USA
[1] 907 Brookside Court, Manchester, CT 06042.
* Corresponding author.
E-mail address: powell@payerprovider.com

Child Adolesc Psychiatric Clin N Am 26 (2017) 125–133
http://dx.doi.org/10.1016/j.chc.2016.07.013
1056-4993/17/© 2016 Elsevier Inc. All rights reserved.

childpsych.theclinics.com

ownership rate of 97%. Furthermore, the study found that most patients were interested in using a mobile application (app) to monitor their mental condition.[2]

Because of their ubiquity, mobile tools provide a potential channel for addressing the mental health needs of adolescents. Adolescents have a particularly strong need for mental health interventions, as roughly half of lifetime mental disorders start by the midteens, and three-quarters by the mid-20s.[3] At the end of adolescence, mental disorders are prevalent, with 52.4% of people aged 18 to 29 experiencing any disorder, and 22.3% experiencing 3 or more disorders. Within this age group, anxiety disorders are most common (30.2%) followed by impulse control disorders (26.8%).[4] Given the high prevalence of smartphone ownership and mental disorders among adolescents, mobile tools for mental health have the potential to expand access to care and lower the cost of care for this critical population.

Two distinct types of mobile tools can be used to provide care: mobile apps, which do not require significant clinician involvement and telepsychiatry tools, which link a patient to a clinician. Mobile tele–mental health has been defined "as the use of mobile phones and other wireless devices as applied to psychiatric and mental health practice."[5] Mobile apps can deliver interactive content, collect information, inform users about insights based on findings, and enable users to receive assistance when in crisis. Furthermore, mobile and computer-based tools can be used to facilitate telepsychiatry interactions, in which a user engages in a videochat with a psychiatrist or other mental health professional.

Because there is somewhat limited available scientific research on the efficacy of smartphone apps in addressing mental disorders, it is difficult to fully characterize their return on investment (ROI).[6] Nonetheless, many are likely to be efficacious, as they are either based on well-proven psychometric instruments (like the Patient Health Questionnaire 9 [PHQ-9]) or are similar to Web-based tools, which have undergone more extensive testing. Web-based tools for cognitive behavioral therapy are found to be effective labor-saving mechanisms for helping patients[7] and for training clinicians to help them.[8,9] Just as many Web-based mental health tools were previously desktop software programs, tools that are currently on the Web are being translated into apps. It is likely that the tools will maintain their effectiveness across platforms, as they are built on common principles.

This article qualitatively describes the sources of direct and indirect benefits of mobile apps for mental health and telepsychiatry. Direct (hard) and indirect (soft) benefit impacts are commonly considered in ROI analyses and differ in that direct benefits result from the immediate expenditures and benefits tied to a good or service, whereas indirect benefits result from the activities and changes that are caused by the good or service.[10] By examining the direct and indirect changes in benefits resulting from these tools, the article identifies key measures that can be quantified by subsequent researchers to gauge their return on investment. The sources of direct and indirect benefits of these tools are summarized in **Table 1** and then discussed in the remainder of the article. This article then provides a methodology for evaluating the ROI of mobile apps and telepsychiatry services and summarizes why such analyses have the potential to facilitate the dissemination of these technologies.

MOBILE APPS FOR MENTAL HEALTH

Mobile apps for mental health provide numerous direct and indirect benefits. The nature of the benefits they provide varies by app, and different users will likely receive different benefits as a result of their app use. As mobile apps typically do not require their users to disclose their identities to make an appointment or to obtain a referral

Table 1 Sources of direct and indirect benefits resulting from digital tools for mental health		
	Mobile Apps for Mental Health	**Telepsychiatry**
Direct	• Savings from substitution for other forms of care • Savings from prevention of higher-acuity situations through early identification and recognition • Increased demand for psychiatric services • Revenue for app developers and operators	• Increased earnings by psychiatrists owing to higher utilization of services • Decreased costs for patients resulting from increased market competition facilitated by the removal of geographic barriers • Decreased transportation costs • Decreased operating costs for psychiatrists • Increased earnings by psychiatrists owing to fewer missed appointments
Indirect	• Savings from better physical health • Increased earnings and economic output from better current performance at work • Increased earnings and economic output from better future performance at work owing to early identification and recognition	• Savings from better physical health • Increased earnings and economic output from better current performance at work • Increased earnings and economic output from better future performance at work owing to early identification and recognition • Decreased lost wages and economic productivity for caregivers

before receiving assistance, they enable users to more easily overcome the inertia that may be preventing them from seeking help. Apps can act as a substitute for live therapy, as an on ramp to live therapy, or as a complement to live therapy. The extent to which apps are a substitute for the labor of mental health professionals depends on the manner in which they are used. When apps enable people to discover that they are in need of help, they may even increase the demand for assistance from clinicians.

Direct Benefits of Mobile Applications for Mental Health

The direct benefits of mobile apps for mental health are savings from substitution for other forms of care, savings from the prevention of higher-acuity situations through early identification and recognition, the creation of demand for psychiatric services as a result of early identification and recognition, and revenue for app developers. Content delivered through apps is less expensive than content delivered by a live person. Building an app has a high sunk cost but little to no incremental cost. As a result, apps can be used as a substitute for labor, particularly in situations in which the labor is repetitive. One National Institute of Mental Health–funded, multisite study showed that traditional cognitive behavioral therapy (CBT) with 16.6 hours of therapist time was equally effective at reducing depression scores as a combination of a computerized CBT program with one-third (5.5 hours) the therapist time.[11] By prerecording basic instruction in CBT, it is possible to eliminate much of the time that therapists spend on repetitive tasks and to instead have them focus on discussions that are specific to the patient. In the case of the aforementioned study, the substitution reduced the cost of CBT by two-thirds. Similar results have been found in education, in which tutored video instruction was found to produce superior outcomes relative to purely live classroom instruction.[12]

An additional direct benefit of mobile apps for mental health is that they can prevent the development of higher-acuity situations. Given the anonymity and convenience surrounding downloading an app, people who would not consider seeking psychiatric assessment by a person may be willing to complete diagnostic questionnaires administered by an app. For instance, there are apps that provide people with the ability to take, log, and trend scores for the PHQ-9[13] and the Generalized Anxiety Disorder 7-Item Scale (GAD-7).[14] The availability of these tools expands access to care by improving access for people uncomfortable seeking live assistance. The US Preventive Services Task Force has recommended the screening of all adults for depression, and app-based screening is one way that this recommendation can be extended to people without good access to care and to adolescents who may be concerned that their responses to a screening will not be handled confidentially.[15] Since children and adolescents are typically not able to obtain live therapeutic help without the assistance of a parent or caregiver, apps play an even more important role in enabling confidential early recognition for this population. Early recognition of depression through apps may be helpful in preventing higher-acuity and costlier problems from developing. Although mild depression can be treated on an outpatient basis, the cost of treating major depression can be far higher, especially if there is a need for inpatient care.

Other parties also directly benefit from apps. Self-identification of mental illness using mobile apps may drive some people to seek assistance from a professional. Many apps, such as those whose only purpose is to administer the GAD-7 or PHQ-9, identify issues but do not provide assistance in solving them,[13,14] which it increases demand for psychiatric services. As apps are often supported by advertising revenue, fees for purchase, or fees for use, they likewise provide a source of revenue to their developers and operators.

Indirect Benefits of Mobile Apps for Mental Health

There are numerous indirect benefits to the early recognition and treatment of mental health issues through mobile apps. Poor mental health can lead to poor physical health, which has its own set of associated costs. Likewise, mental health issues can impact present performance at school and at work, as well as future performance at work.

Mental health conditions can lead to increased costs related to physical health, as mental health conditions increase the risk of communicable and noncommunicable disease.[16] Although many chronic conditions do not manifest until after adolescence, early recognition and treatment of mental illness have the potential to improve subsequent physical health outcomes. Findings show that people with diabetes and mental health conditions are less likely to meet diabetes performance measures. Namely, they are less likely to receive hemoglobin A1c testing, to receive low-density lipoprotein cholesterol testing, to receive an eye examination, to have glycemic control, and to have lipemic control.[17] In addition to increasing physical health care costs, mental health conditions can cause a loss of economic productivity by increasing mortality. The presence of depression and other mental health conditions are found to increase the rate of mortality after a person experiences a stroke.[18]

Mental health conditions affect how adolescents perform both inside and outside the classroom. Higher scores on the Children's Depression Inventory among adolescents referred for behavioral treatment of recurrent headache are associated with higher school absenteeism and lower academic performance.[19] Likewise, depression adversely affects the academic performance of university students.[20,21] High school performance affects college admissions, and college selectivity is found to affect future earnings.[22] In adults, depression is associated with multiple types of presenteeism (presence at work with reduced productivity caused by health-related impairment): limitations in time management, issues with interpersonal functioning, and overall output.[23] These losses in productivity impact both the individual and the society in which he or she lives, as society benefits from the taxation and resale of productive work. Given that mobile apps can be used to diagnose and treat depression, they have the potential to reduce its present and future financial consequences.

TELEPSYCHIATRY

Telepsychiatry offers greater convenience to the patient and the psychiatrist. As a result, direct and indirect benefits can accrue to both parties from the participation in telepsychiatry sessions. Like mobile applications, telepsychiatry sessions can serve as an on ramp, substitute, or complement to traditional care. Psychiatrists can devote themselves fully to telepsychiatry or use it as a means for supplementing their incomes while widening their reach, enabling them to connect with remote patients.

Direct Benefits of Telepsychiatry

Patients benefit from telepsychiatry, in that it increases access to psychiatric care while potentially lowering costs.[24,25] By removing geographic barriers to access, it makes mental health services more accessible in rural areas and to bedbound or agoraphobic people.[26] Furthermore, when patients receive care at home (which is not always the case), it eliminates the cost of transportation associated with the office visit. Removing transportation from care also lowers both the monetary and time cost of attending a session. This makes psychiatry more accessible to people with limited time, income, or access to transportation. In doing so, it increases the likelihood that people in remote areas will have adequate access to care and to obtain the benefits that it provides. Even people who do not live in remote areas have the potential to benefit, as telepsychiatry can enable them to have greater continuity of care while traveling. Psychiatrists providing telepsychiatry services from home can also save on the cost of transportation.

Services offering instant access to a psychiatrist may increase the ability of patients to receive help at times of urgent need, whether at home, traveling, or in a clinical setting without ready access to a psychiatrist. A survey found that primary care physicians referring children and adolescents for telepsychiatry are satisfied with the care delivered and believe that it makes psychiatric consultations more available to patients.[27] Although psychiatry on demand may be less beneficial if used on a regular basis, it may be a helpful supplement to patients unable to reach their usual clinician while in a time of need. Suicide hotlines provide people with effective immediate assistance.[28] Telepsychiatry services have the potential to provide an enhanced version of such access.

The convenience of telepsychiatry additionally has profound benefits for the psychiatrist. Telepsychiatry services expand the market reach of a clinician, providing a greater number of potential patients to fill a schedule. Furthermore, telepsychiatry patients may be less likely to miss appointments, as transportation is no longer a barrier to attendance.[29] Telepsychiatry services may likewise be able to fill holes in a psychiatrist's calendar arising from last-minute cancellations. As a result, psychiatrists can increase their utilization. Although concerns remain over reimbursement for telepsychiatry sessions,[30] to the extent that they can be used to fill unscheduled time, they may enable psychiatrists to increase revenues while enabling patients to access care at a lower total cost. While the payment arrangement between the health insurer, the health system, and the psychiatrist determines who ultimately captures the benefit of the increased capacity, a benefit exists whenever the additional capacity is put to productive use. Psychiatrists paid by the session can increase their incomes, and salaried psychiatrists can increase the capacities of their facilities, enabling them to treat larger numbers of patients.

Indirect Benefits of Telepsychiatry

In addition to providing direct benefits, telepsychiatry provides indirect benefits to patients and their caregivers. Telepsychiatric appointments reduce the need for a caregiver to assist the patient in attending the appointment, lowering the costs that appointment attendance imposes on third parties.[31] Since most children and adolescents need someone to transport them to the office of a psychiatrist, it is more likely that there will be a burden on caregivers than is the case in the treatment of adult patients.

The implications of a patient encounter that does not involve the use of an office can lead to multiple forms of savings for psychiatrists purely engaging in telepsychiatric practice. Psychiatrists can save money on staff and office space, as telepsychiatric appointments do not require the use of a physical waiting room or the completion of paper forms. Eliminating the physical visit eliminates the need to insure against some of the liabilities that such a visit may produce (eg, slips and falls). When no office is used, the psychiatrist saves on staffing, utilities, waiting room items (eg, water, magazines, and tissues), and furnishings (eg, couches, antique rugs, lamps). Although equipment is required for telepsychiatry, laptops with cameras, smartphones, and broadband connections have recently become so ubiquitous that it is increasingly unlikely that many psychiatrists will experience incremental equipment costs.

Telepsychiatry produces the same indirect benefits as mobile apps. To the extent that telepsychiatry improves mental health, it has the potential to improve grades in school, present earnings, and future earnings. Likewise, as mental illness amplifies the costs associated with physical illness, telepsychiatry has the potential to lead to savings on somatic medicine.

AREAS FOR FUTURE EXPLORATION

Although there is substantial evidence to suggest that mobile apps and telemedicine are effective methods of addressing mental health demand and that there are substantial costs to untreated mental illness, there is sparse research on the ROI of these digital interventions. Additional assessments and evaluations of the impact of specific tools on specific mental health conditions are also needed. Future research likely needs to focus on sizing specific direct or indirect benefits resulting from specific tools. The benefits highlighted in **Table 1** likely need to each be explored in the context of specific tool/illness pairs. Some benefits will not be disease specific, such as reduced transportation costs or office overhead associated with telepsychiatry. Other benefits, such as the savings on care for physical health, will be disease specific. Costs will differ between interventions and will be highly dependent on how they are implemented. For instance, some psychiatrists will completely devote themselves to home-based telepsychiatry, eliminating the need for an office, whereas others will engage in telepsychiatry while in a formal office setting and will not be able to eliminate office-related costs. Likewise, the presence of value-based contracts will determine whether health insurance companies will incur additional expenses as a consequence of increased demand for psychiatry. Value-based contracts also affect how financial benefits accrue to the psychiatrist.

> **Box 1**
> **Health care return on investment analysis framework**
>
> - Who pays directly and indirectly, and how much?
> - Who benefits directly and indirectly, and how much?
> - When do the benefits and costs arrive?
> - What are the probabilities that the benefits and costs will exist?
>
> *Adapted* from Payer+Provider Syndicate. ROI Analysis. Available at: http://payerprovider.com/roi-analysis/. Accessed June 27, 2016.

Regardless of the intervention or disease being examined, a common set of questions can be studied to determine direct and indirect benefits and costs. The questions shown in **Box 1** can be used to identify the key variables that impact the ROI of a health care innovation. The process of understanding ROI begins by listing all of the sources of benefit and cost associated with an intervention. Some benefits and costs will not initially have a monetary value, such as health improvements or time savings. For the purposes of calculation, all values can be denominated in currency. Health improvements can be converted into currency units by making assumptions about the value that the society in question places on a quality-adjusted life-year. Likewise, time savings for an employer can be valued using estimates of labor productivity, and time savings for employees can be valued using estimates of wages. In calculating the ROI, it is also important to consider the timing of benefits and costs and the probabilities that they will exist. It may be necessary to calculate both short-term and long-term estimates of ROI, as some investors may be uninterested in interventions that provide a positive ROI in the long run but not in the short run. Since many interventions do not affect everyone who uses them and may also not receive uptake from everyone who is offered them, it is necessary to consider the probabilities that each of the benefits and costs examined will ultimately materialize.

SUMMARY

Smartphone use is nearly universal among adolescents. Smartphones are available to most adolescents of all ages, races, and levels of household income. As mental illness often develops during adolescence, and adolescents may have issues accessing care because of cost, lack of transportation, or lack of independence, mental health services delivered via smartphones have the potential to significantly and positively impact these populations. Mobile applications for mental health and telepsychiatry services reduce many of the barriers to receiving a diagnosis or treatment. In doing so, they generate a series of direct and indirect benefits. Adolescents may benefit in the short term with improved psychological wellbeing, and these short-term improvements may have a long-run impact on overall health and workplace productivity. Even clinicians stand to gain from these technologies, as they have the potential to reduce costs and increase revenue. Although the benefits of mobile apps and telepsychiatry services have yet to be adequately characterized, the increasing ubiquity of these tools has created a call to action for doing so. As the ROI of these powerful tools becomes clearer, they may gain increasing support from both clinicians and managed care organizations. Demonstrating the value of these tools may help them become a part of mainstream care, benefiting more people with unmet needs, including the highly vulnerable adolescent population.

DISCLOSURES

A.C. Powell is President of the health care consulting firm Payer+Provider Syndicate, a member of the Scientific Advisory Board of PsyberGuide, and a member of the Editorial Board of the *Journal of Medical Internet Research: Mental Health*. He has received salary from Payer+Provider Syndicate for evaluating the return on investment of health care innovations, and has received fees from PsyberGuide for evaluating digital tools for mental health. M. Chen is the CEO of VSee Lab, a telehealth company creating the software and hardware for telehealth implementations. He is paid by VSee Lab. C. Thammachart is a third-year medical student at the University of New England. She consults for IBM in the development of Watson Radiology technology and services.

REFERENCES

1. Lernhart A. A majority of American teens report access to a computer, game console, smartphone, and a tablet. Pew Research Center. Available at: http://www.pewinternet.org/2015/04/09/a-majority-of-american-teens-report-access-to-a-computer-game-console-smartphone-and-a-tablet/. Accessed May 27, 2016.
2. Torous J, Friedman R, Keshavan M. Smartphone ownership and interest in mobile applications to monitor symptoms of mental health conditions. JMIR Mhealth Uhealth 2014;2(1):e2.
3. Kessler RC, Amminger GP, Aguilar-gaxiola S, et al. Age of onset of mental disorders: a review of recent literature. Curr Opin Psychiatry 2007;20(4):359–64.
4. Kessler RC, Berglund P, Demler O, et al. Lifetime prevalence and age-of-onset distributions of DSM-IV disorders in the National Comorbidity Survey Replication. Arch Gen Psychiatry 2005;62(6):593–602.
5. Chan SR, Torous J, Hinton L, et al. Mobile tele-mental health: increasing applications and a move to hybrid models of care. Healthcare 2014;2(2):220–33.
6. Torous J, Powell AC. Current research and trends in the use of smartphone applications for mood disorders. Internet Interventions 2015;2(2):169–73.
7. Wright JH, Wright AS, Albano AM, et al. Computer-assisted cognitive therapy for depression: maintaining efficacy while reducing therapist time. Am J Psychiatry 2005;162(6):1158–64.
8. McDonough M, Marks IM. Teaching medical students exposure therapy for phobia/panic–randomized, controlled comparison of face-to-face tutorial in small groups vs. solo computer instruction. Med Educ 2002;36(5):412–7.
9. Gega L, Norman IJ, Marks IM. Computer-aided vs. tutor-delivered teaching of exposure therapy for phobia/panic: randomized controlled trial with pre-registration nursing students. Int J Nurs Stud 2007;44(3):397–405.
10. Health Resources & Services Administration. What return on investment (ROI) models can I use. Available at: http://www.hrsa.gov/healthit/toolbox/Rural HealthITtoolbox/Financing/roi.html. Accessed June 27, 2016.
11. Wright JH, Brown G, Eels T, et al. Computer-assisted cognitive-behavioral therapy for depression: acute treatment phase outcome. Poster Presented at the National Network of Depression Centers Annual Meeting. Chicago, October 22-24, 2014.
12. Gibbons JF, Kincheloe WR, Down KS. Tutored videotape instruction: a new use of electronics media in education. Science 1977;195(4283):1139–46.
13. iTunes App Store. STAT Depression Screening PHQ-9. Apple. Available at: https://itunes.apple.com/us/app/stat-depression-screening/id348793894?mt=8. Accessed May 29, 2016.

14. iTunes App Store. GAD-7 Anxiety Scale. Apple. Available at: https://itunes.apple.com/us/app/gad-7-anxiety-scale/id587189044?mt=8. Accessed May 29, 2016.
15. Siu AL, Bibbins-domingo K, Grossman DC, et al. Screening for depression in adults: US preventive services task Force recommendation statement. JAMA 2016;315(4):380–7.
16. Prince M, Patel V, Saxena S, et al. No health without mental health. Lancet 2007; 370(9590):859–77.
17. Frayne SM, Halanych JH, Miller DR, et al. Disparities in diabetes care: impact of mental illness. Arch Intern Med 2005;165(22):2631–8.
18. Williams LS, Ghose SS, Swindle RW. Depression and other mental health diagnoses increase mortality risk after ischemic stroke. Am J Psychiatry 2004;161(6): 1090–5.
19. Breuner CC, Smith MS, Womack WM. Factors related to school absenteeism in adolescents with recurrent headache. Headache 2004;44(3):217–22.
20. Heiligenstein E, Guenther G, Hsu K, et al. Depression and academic impairment in college students. J Am Coll Health 1996;45(2):59–64.
21. Hysenbegasi A, Hass SL, Rowland CR. The impact of depression on the academic productivity of university students. J Ment Health Policy Econ 2005;8(3): 145.
22. Loury LD, Garman D. College selectivity and earnings. J Labor Econ 1995;289–308.
23. Burton WN, Pransky G, Conti DJ, et al. The association of medical conditions and presenteeism. J Occup Environ Med 2004;46(6):S38–45.
24. Wade VA, Karnon J, Elshaug AG, et al. A systematic review of economic analyses of telehealth services using real time video communication. BMC Health Serv Res 2010;10:233.
25. Hyler SE, Gangure DP. A review of the costs of telepsychiatry. Psychiatr Serv 2003;54(7):976–80.
26. Brown FW. Rural telepsychiatry. Psychiatr Serv 1998;49(7):963–4.
27. Myers KM, Valentine JM, Melzer SM. Feasibility, acceptability, and sustainability of telepsychiatry for children and adolescents. Psychiatr Serv 2007;58(11): 1493–6.
28. Rhee WK, Merbaum M, Strube MJ, et al. Efficacy of brief telephone psychotherapy with callers to a suicide hotline. Suicide Life Threat Behav 2005;35(3): 317–28.
29. Glueck DA. Telepsychiatry in private practice. Child Adolesc Psychiatr Clin N Am 2011;20(1):1–11.
30. Deslich S, Stec B, Tomblin S, et al. Telepsychiatry in the 21(st) century: transforming healthcare with technology. Perspect Health Inf Manag 2013;10:1f.
31. Spaulding R, Belz N, Delurgio S, et al. Cost savings of telemedicine utilization for child psychiatry in a rural Kansas community. Telemed J E Health 2010;16(8): 867–71.

Index

Note: Page numbers of article titles are in **boldface** type.

Child Adolesc Psychiatric Clin N Am 26 (2017) 135–141
http://dx.doi.org/10.1016/S1056-4993(16)30108-0
1056-4993/17

Moving?

Make sure your subscription moves with you!

To notify us of your new address, find your **Clinics Account Number** (located on your mailing label above your name), and contact customer service at:

Email: journalscustomerservice-usa@elsevier.com

800-654-2452 (subscribers in the U.S. & Canada)
314-447-8871 (subscribers outside of the U.S. & Canada)

Fax number: 314-447-8029

Elsevier Health Sciences Division
Subscription Customer Service
3251 Riverport Lane
Maryland Heights, MO 63043

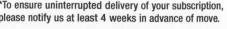

*To ensure uninterrupted delivery of your subscription, please notify us at least 4 weeks in advance of move.

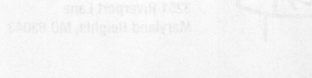

Printed and bound by CPI Group (UK) Ltd, Croydon, CR0 4YY

12/10/2024

01773485-0002